Enjoying Food Peace

Recipes and Intuitive Eating Wisdom to Nourish Your Body and Mind

Bonnie R. Giller, MS, RDN, CDN, CDE

The information in this book is for informational and educational purposes only. It is not intended as a substitute for professional medical advice or the care of a physician. Do not use this information to diagnose or treat a health problem or disease. If you suspect you have a health problem, please contact your health care provider.

Copyright © 2019 Bonnie R. Giller, MS, RDN, CDN, CDE
All rights reserved.
ISBN-13: 978-0-578-46004-8
Book design by Samantha Baturin

To my husband, Michael, for always believing in me and cheering me on to achieve my goals and dreams.

To my children, Matthew and Shaina, Jason and Shira, Jennifer and Lauren for your willingness to taste test recipes and for giving me your honest opinion when I needed to go back to the drawing board.

To my grandsons, Evan and Zach, who always put a smile on my face!

To my parents, Ruth and Danny Berger. There are no words to express how grateful I am for all you have taught me and for being my guiding light in life and in business. Thank you, thank you, thank you!

To my clients, who give me the inspiration to continue to create new products and services. Your nutrition questions and thirst for knowledge gives me the motivation to keep on doing what I love. Thank you.

And last, but not least, thank you to my assistant Samantha Baturin. Samantha had a creative vision for this book and took that vision and made it a reality. Many thanks for all the hours you spent formatting and designing the book. You are one of a kind!

Radiant Reviews for Enjoying Food Peace

"It was so refreshing to dive into a cookbook with not only delicious recipes but also full of intuitive eating and body wisdom sprinkled throughout. Intuitive eating is about making peace with food which opens you up to new possibility with cooking."

    Angela Prior LCSW, RYT, Licensed Clinical Social Worker
    Certified Intuitive Eating Counselor

"The recipes and gentle guidance in this book are a great reminder for our diet-obsessed culture that food can actually be pleasurable and sustaining, both physically and psychologically. We don't have to sacrifice emotional wellness in the name of nutrition. We were born knowing how to have both, at the same time, bite by bite."

    Kyrie Russ, MS, Licensed Clinical Professional Counselor
    Certified Intuitive Eating Counselor

"*Enjoying Food Peace* offers delicious recipes topped off with a helpful serving of the Intuitive Eating principles. With each chapter, Bonnie shares tidbits to help readers enjoy their food and pass on any diet guilt!"

    Kim Hoban, RDN, CDN, CPT
    Registered Dietitian, KH Nutrition

"It's been said we 'eat with our eyes' first; however, *Enjoying Food Peace* entice the reader's mind from the start with over 150 recipes full of combinations of textures, colors and flavor that inspire the palette. As a Registered Dietitian and Certified Intuitive Eating Counselor I often am looking for a way to introduce the concept of "gentle nutrition" to clients while avoiding the diet mentality messages that accompany a lot of recipe blogs and cookbooks. Bonnie Giller has bridged that gap with *Enjoying Food Peace*. It is a beautiful compilation of recipes using commonly-sourced whole food ingredients and easy to follow directions – interspersed with wisdom reinforcing an intuitive eating approach. A great resource for preparing and enjoying nutritious meals at home!"

    Holly Paulsen, RD, CEDRD, LD
    Certified Registered Eating Disorders Dietitian and Certified Intuitive Eating Counselor

Table of Contents

1 | Introduction
5 | Essential Broths
9 | Soups
33 | Salads
53 | Dips & Dressings
71 | Hot Sides
103 | Cold Sides
125 | Kugels & Latkes
143 | Poultry & Meat
181 | Fish
205 | Dairy & Pasta Entrees
221 | Vegetarian
239 | Breakfast
251 | Muffins & Breads
269 | Desserts
291 | Appendix

Introduction

Imagine if you had all the money you have ever spent on diet programs. What could you buy? Diamond earrings, a gold watch, a new car, a summer home? Think back to those diet programs. While they worked for you short-term, what happened after you went off the diet? More than likely, the pounds you lost returned with a few bonus pounds as well. You see, most diets will work at first because when you cut calories, you will lose weight. That's just science! The problem most people face is that they fail to make lifelong behavioral changes and that is why the weight comes back.

Now think about the reason you started each diet program. Maybe you were preparing for a wedding, your high school reunion, or some other big event. The appeal of dieting is that it's fairly easy to follow a set of rules or pre-planned menus and see immediate results. The problem is that diets do not address the habits that caused you to put on weight in the first place. That's why after following diet rules for a certain period of time, you eventually gain back the weight you lost. Whether that big event you were dieting for passes or you were triggered by an emotional upset, a major life change, or work stress that has you reaching for comfort food, eventually the diet comes to an end and the old eating habits and weight return.

Truthfully, no form of dieting is going to work for losing weight and keeping it off. For the more than three decades that I've been in private practice, I have told my clients that I don't "do diets". Diet is a "four letter word" that is not to be used in my office. I have created countless customized meal plans for people specific to their nutritional needs, have counseled on behavior modification techniques and strategies, and worked with them on changing their eating habits to improve their health. While this approach has helped many clients, I also noticed that many people were taking their meal plans and using them as just another diet or set of rules instructing them on when to eat and how much to eat. I knew there must be another way to help individuals struggling with going on and off every diet. That is when I discovered *intuitive eating*.

Intuitive eating is characterized by eating based on your physiological hunger and satiety (fullness) cues rather than situational and emotional cues. Every individual is born with the natural instinct to know when they are hungry and when they are satisfied enough to stop eating. Think of a newborn baby who cries when they are hungry and will push away when they are full. Oftentimes, well-meaning parents are inclined to say "they didn't finish their bottle; they didn't eat enough" and will try to feed the baby a little more, having them push away again. When the baby becomes a bit older and sits in a high chair, adults use tricks and games like "flying" the spoon through the air to get the baby to eat more. Then as toddlers, they run around playing, not wanting to sit to eat lunch. While you may worry that they will go hungry, in fact children are simply exhibiting what is natural to them: the innate ability to eat when hungry and to stop when full.

What happens over the years as you become an adult that strips you of this ability?

Maybe you can look back on your childhood and remember being encouraged to "clean your plate" if you wanted dessert or to tidy your room if you wanted to go out for a treat of ice cream. These tactics all go against the natural ability to tune into your hunger and satiety cues. As you got older, your recognition of these signals were destroyed further by the multi-billion dollar diet industry and the fad diets and gimmicks that flood all channels of media.

Intuitive eating bridges the gap that is created over the years, reconnecting you with your body's natural cues. As an intuitive eater, you do not eat out of boredom, loneliness, sadness, happiness, stress, or anxiety. You do not eat because you are at a free buffet or because someone brought cookies to work. You do not eat mindlessly, munching on a bag of chips while watching television. You do not engage in conditioned eating behaviors like plowing through a bucket of popcorn at the movies simply because "that's just what you do at the movies!" As an intuitive eater, you eat when your body signals that you are hungry and need to eat and you stop when you are satisfied.

Everyone has an intuitive eater buried within them. The problem is the urgency to find that magic bullet that will get the weight off now. As a result, you try one diet after another, only to be disappointed when you regain the weight. You end up with very little trust in yourself, your body, and the foods you choose.

I want you to know that if you have struggled with this cycle of dieting, you have not failed. It's the diets that have failed you. The question now is how to change a lifetime of eating habits. How do you reclaim the attunement you were born with? How do you become an intuitive eater again?

Intuitive eating is not a diet or a meal plan. Instead of telling you what or how much to eat, it helps you tune into what is going on in your body and mind. It encourages you to become aware of your emotional, psychological, and physiological motivations to eat. By engaging in intuitive eating, you are better able to balance what you eat, the way you eat, and why you eat.

Introduction

The key to achieving a healthy body you love (without the trials and tribulations of dieting) is learning to combine three essential ingredients: a healthy mindset, caring support, and nutrition education. Balancing these three pieces create the backbone to a loving, nurturing relationship with your body.

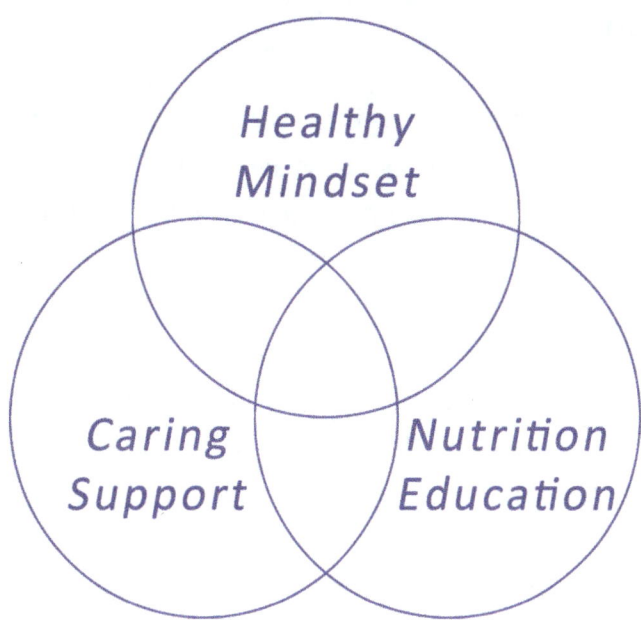

Intuitive eating, an approach to eating created by two Registered Dietitians, Evelyn Tribole and Elyse Resch, encompasses 10 principles which I explain throughout this book. These principles will put you on the path to taking charge of your health, rebuilding trust in yourself and your body, and enjoying a new relationship with food. Intuitive eating is not about restriction or deprivation. Go ahead and eat that piece of cake!

Intuitive eating fosters making peace with food and ditching labeling food as good or bad. This approach helps to create a healthy relationship with food, mind, and body. The benefits of this approach are achieved by exploring how you got to where you are today and understanding where you are headed. Intuitive eating encourages respecting your body and honoring your health. With the 10 principles as a guide, you learn to modify your self-perception to a more realistic view. Honoring your health encourages a consistent progression to improved health by guiding you to nourishing meal options.

My intention for writing this cookbook is to help you understand that it *is* possible to achieve a healthy life and a body you love while eating the foods you love. By utilizing the 3 essential ingredients, you are able to balance intuition and nutrition, make peace with food, and enjoy guilt-free eating all while nourishing your body. Caring for and nourishing your body does not mean depriving yourself of your favorite foods. Instead, the goal is to find balance in your eating, respect for your body, and attunement with your inner signals. Being an intuitive eater gives you the freedom to eat without guilt.

In intuitive eating, nutrition is not ignored. This is often a common misconception, however, it is important to shift out of a diet mentality before considering nutrition. Otherwise, the nutrition information will be heard by you as more diet rules. Once you have rejected the diet mentality and have made peace with food, you will be ready to look at the nutritional value of your food choices.

In intuitive eating, we consider nutrition from a gentle perspective. It's called *Gentle Nutrition*, where you consider nutrition AND taste when making your food choices to honor both your health and your taste buds. Gentle Nutrition Facts for each recipe are included in the appendix of the book for when you are ready to integrate Gentle Nutrition into your intuitive eating life.

As the author of this book and creator of the recipes, I noted that lower fat dairy products produced a better flavor and mouthfeel and felt better in *my* body. However, you might prefer the taste and feel of full fat dairy, so by all means, use the ingredients that feel best for you. Intuitive eating enables you to tune inward and make the food and nutrition decisions that are unique for your body.

There are recipes in the pages that follow that perhaps as a dieter you'd say "I cannot eat that" but as an intuitive eater, you will enjoy! This is not a book filled only with salads, juices, and smoothies, although these are delicious too, but with nourishing meals and surprising twists on some classic favorites.

To get started, I am going to share with you my Essential Chicken and Veggie Broths. These are easy to make and can be used as the foundation for homemade soups, sauces, or any other recipe that calls for broth. Enjoy!

Introduction

BRG Chicken Broth

MAKES 2 QUARTS TOTAL

INGREDIENTS

- 2 (2 ½ - pound) broiler-fryer chickens, skinned and cut into eighths
- 10 cups water
- 6 stalks celery, cut into thirds
- 6 large carrots, cut into thirds
- 2 cloves garlic, minced
- 1 medium onion, cut into quarters
- 3 sprigs fresh thyme
- ¼ teaspoon black pepper

INSTRUCTIONS

1. Put chicken in a large soup pot. Add water and bring to a boil.
2. Add celery, carrots, garlic, onion, and thyme and lower heat.
3. Add black pepper and simmer uncovered for at least 2 hours. Skim impurities off the top of broth with a spoon as necessary.
4. Strain broth into separate container and cool.
5. Use BRG Chicken Broth as a base to your favorite soup recipes.

BRG Veggie Broth

MAKES 1 ½ QUARTS TOTAL

INGREDIENTS

- 1 large sweet onion, cut into quarters
- 3 stalks celery, cut into thirds
- 3 large carrots, cut into thirds
- 2 cloves garlic, minced
- 1 bunch scallions, chopped
- 1 leek, cut in half lengthwise
- ½ cup chopped fresh basil
- 10 cups water
- 2 bay leaves
- ⅛ teaspoon black pepper

INSTRUCTIONS

1. Put onion, celery, carrots, garlic, scallions, leek, and basil in a large soup pot. Add water and bring to a boil.
2. Add bay leaves and black pepper.
3. Reduce to medium-low heat and simmer for approximately 45 minutes to 1 hour.
4. Strain broth into separate container and cool.
5. Use BRG Veggie Broth for a perfect base to all your soups.

Intuitive Eating Wisdom

A healthy mindset gives you unconditional permission to eat what you desire when you are hungry without the worry of overeating. By opening up to the possibility of eating what your body is asking for without stressing over diet rules or restrictions, you are allowing yourself to nourish your body without guilt.

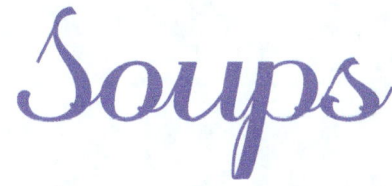

Soups

IN THIS CHAPTER

- 11 | Amazing Artichoke Soup
- 12 | Old-Fashioned Hearty Chicken Soup
- 14 | Roasted Chestnut Soup
- 15 | Chunky Vegetable Soup
- 16 | Sweet & Spicy Carrot Soup
- 18 | Zesty Gazpacho
- 19 | Cream of Broccoli Soup
- 20 | Mexican Squash Soup
- 22 | Creamy Sweet Potato Soup
- 23 | Onion Soup
- 24 | Mushroom Barley Soup
- 26 | Corn Chowder
- 27 | Pasta Fagioli Soup
- 28 | Creamy Tomato Soup with Couscous
- 29 | Strawberries & Crème Soup

Amazing Artichoke Soup

Artichokes are not often a vegetable you'll find highlighted in soup. That's why I'm sure you'll love this! The artichoke hearts are bursting with flavor in every bite and the yogurt is the secret ingredient for a smooth creamy texture.

MAKES 5 SERVINGS

INGREDIENTS

- 1 medium onion, chopped
- 2 cloves garlic, minced
- 1 tablespoon olive oil
- 1 (10-ounce) box frozen artichoke hearts (approximately 9 artichoke hearts)
- 2 ½ cups low sodium vegetable broth
- 1 small potato, peeled and cubed
- 1 cup chopped frozen or fresh spinach
- ½ tablespoon dried thyme
- ¼ teaspoon salt
- ½ cup plain nonfat yogurt

INSTRUCTIONS

1. In a soup pot, sauté onions and garlic in olive oil.
2. Add artichoke hearts and broth. Bring to a boil, then reduce to a simmer.
3. Add potato, spinach, thyme, and salt.
4. Return to a boil, then reduce to medium-low heat. Cover and cook for 45 minutes or until vegetables are soft.
5. Remove from heat and puree using an immersion or free-standing blender.
6. Stir in yogurt and heat through.

Old-Fashioned Hearty Chicken Soup

When I think of visiting my grandparents as a child, I can recall the smell of chicken soup on the stove. This soup brings back those wonderful memories of family times. It will warm your soul and satisfy your taste buds.

MAKES 8 SERVINGS

INGREDIENTS

- 4 pounds broiler-fryer chicken, skinned and cut into eighths
- 12 cups water (approximately 3 quarts)
- 3 stalks celery, cut into halves
- 3 large carrots, cut into thirds
- 2 cloves garlic, minced
- 1 medium onion, cut into fourths
- 1 turnip, cut into fourths
- 1 leek, cut in half lengthwise
- ½ bunch fresh parsley
- ½ bunch fresh dill
- 1 teaspoon salt
- ¼ teaspoon black pepper

INSTRUCTIONS

1. Put chicken in a large soup pot. Add water and bring to a boil.
2. Add celery, carrots, garlic, onion, turnip, leek, parsley, and dill and lower heat.
3. Add salt and black pepper and simmer for approximately 1 hour. Skim impurities off the top of soup with a spoon as necessary.
4. Chill in refrigerator overnight. Skim any remaining fat off the top before reheating.

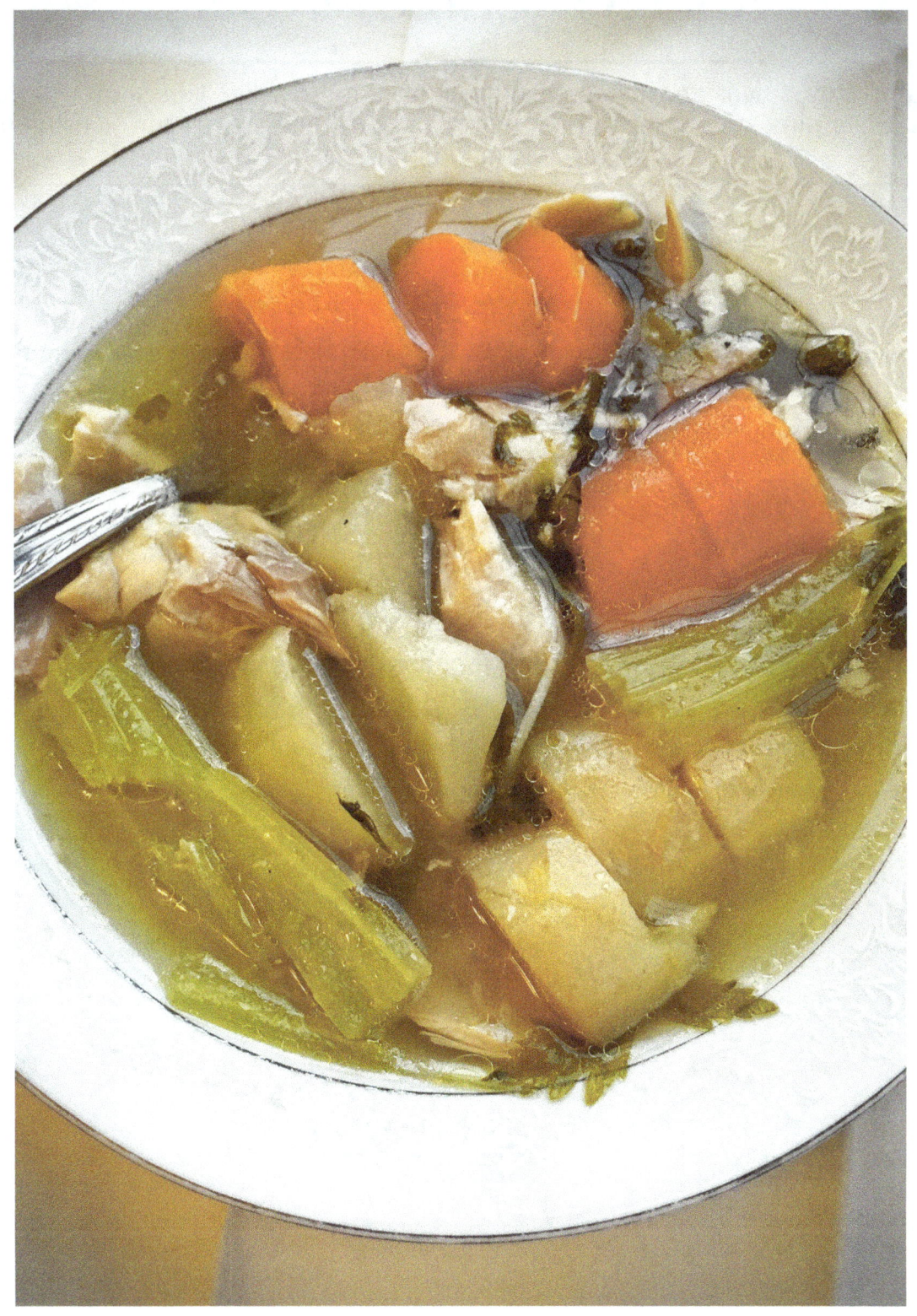

Roasted Chestnut Soup

You know how smells and flavors can bring back memories? This soup will do just that. Chestnuts are not a common ingredient but they are certain to bring back the joys of the holiday season.

MAKES 15 SERVINGS

INGREDIENTS

- 4 medium onions, chopped (approximately 2 cups)
- 14 stalks celery, chopped (approximately 7 cups)
- 1 teaspoon olive oil
- 3 quarts low sodium vegetable broth
- 20-ounces roasted chestnuts (approximately 4 bags)
- Garlic powder, to taste

INSTRUCTIONS

1. In a soup pot, sauté onions and celery in olive oil for 10 minutes until soft and translucent.
2. Add vegetable broth and bring to a boil.
3. Add chestnuts and garlic powder. Cook uncovered 1 ½ hours until chestnuts are soft.
4. Puree with an immersion blender or free-standing blender.

Soups

Chunky Vegetable Soup

Just a little slicing and dicing and ta-da, you have a satisfying nutritious soup! It will give you essential vitamins and minerals to keep you feeling your best. The blend of spices and herbs are perfect to make the vegetables burst with flavor.

MAKES 14 SERVINGS

INGREDIENTS

- 1 medium onion, diced
- 2 cloves garlic, chopped
- 1 cup sliced fresh mushrooms
- 2 stalks celery, sliced
- 3 carrots, chopped
- 3 large tomatoes, diced
- 1 medium green bell pepper, diced
- 1 (8-ounce) can crushed tomatoes
- 1 cup chopped cabbage
- 1 cup fresh green beans
- 1 cup broccoli florets
- 5 cups low sodium vegetable broth
- 2 cups water
- ½ tablespoon oregano
- 1 tablespoon chopped fresh parsley
- 2 tablespoons basil
- 1 tablespoon thyme
- ⅛ teaspoon black pepper

INSTRUCTIONS

1. Combine all ingredients in a soup pot.
2. Bring to a boil, then lower the heat. Cover and simmer until vegetables are tender, approximately 45 minutes.

Sweet & Spicy Carrot Soup

With yellow raisins and brown sugar, this soup will satisfy your taste buds and leave you wanting more. Pair this with a black bean salad and you have a perfect wholesome meal.

MAKES 7 SERVINGS

INGREDIENTS

- 6 cups low sodium vegetable broth
- 2 pounds carrots, peeled and sliced
- ¼ teaspoon ground cumin
- 1 tablespoon brown sugar
- 1 cup plain soy milk
- ¼ teaspoon salt
- ¼ cup golden raisins
- 1 tablespoon chopped dill

INSTRUCTIONS

1. In a soup pot, bring vegetable broth to a boil.
2. Add carrots, cumin, brown sugar, soy milk, and salt. Bring to a boil, then lower to medium-low heat and cook for 45 minutes.
3. Remove from heat and let cool slightly. Using an immersion or free-standing blender, blend until smooth.
4. Mix in raisins and dill. Heat and serve.

Soups

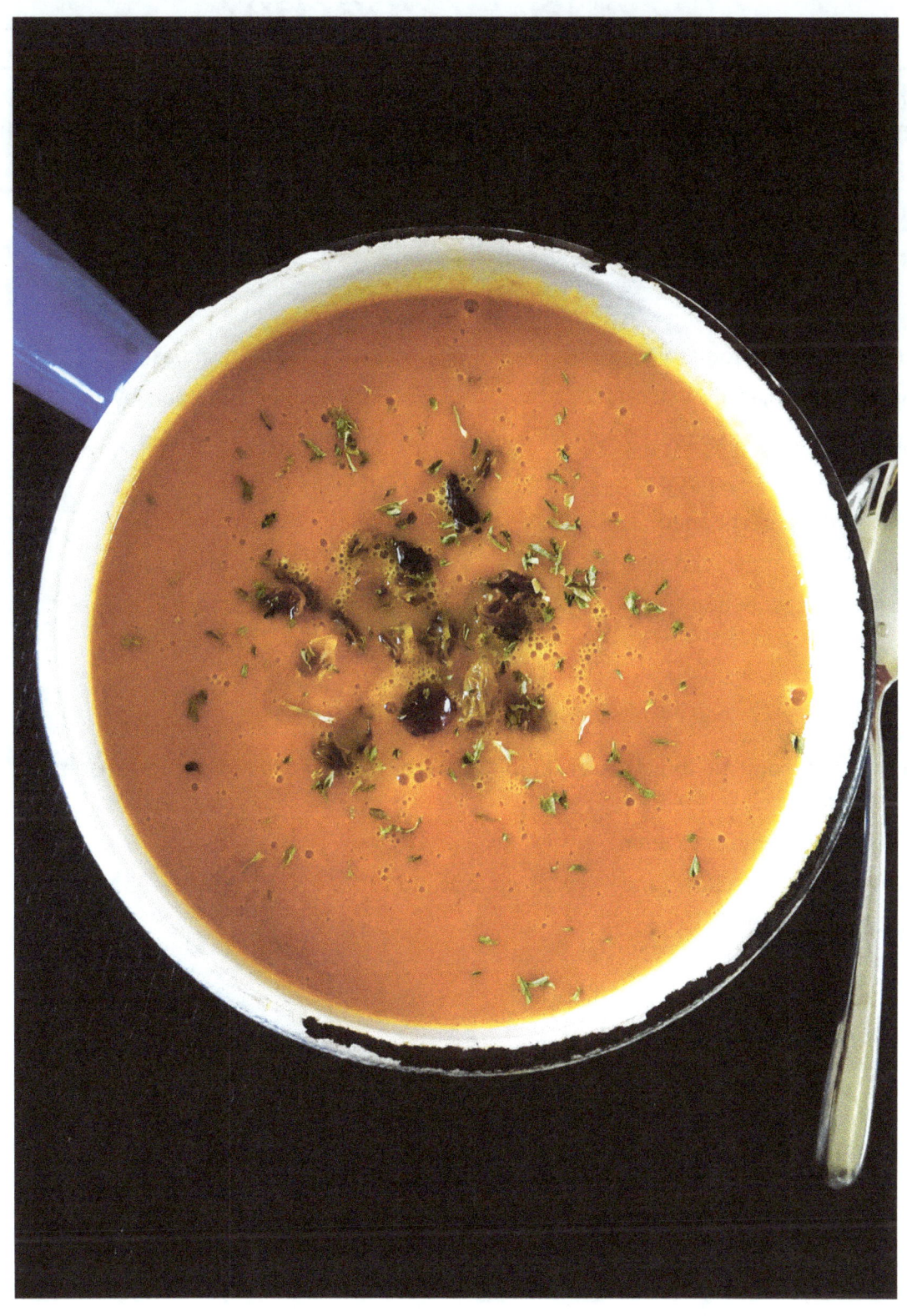

Zesty Gazpacho

Too hot to enjoy soup during the spring and summer months? Not anymore! You'll find this cool, flavorful soup to be a refreshing and unique appetizer in the warmer months.

MAKES 9 SERVINGS

INGREDIENTS

- 4 cups low sodium tomato juice
- 1 medium onion, diced
- 2 large tomatoes, chopped
- 1 green bell pepper, chopped
- 1 red bell pepper, chopped
- 1 medium cucumber, chopped
- 2 cloves garlic, chopped
- ¼ cup chopped fresh basil
- ¼ cup chopped fresh parsley
- ¼ teaspoon ground cumin
- 1 avocado, diced
- 2 tablespoons lemon juice
- 2 tablespoons red wine vinegar
- 2 drops Tabasco Sauce (optional)

INSTRUCTIONS

1. In a soup pot, combine tomato juice, onion, tomatoes, green and red pepper, cucumber, and garlic and mix well.
2. Stir in basil, parsley, and cumin.
3. Add avocado, lemon juice, and red wine vinegar. Add Tabasco sauce if desired.
4. Chill for at least 2 hours and serve.

Cream of Broccoli Soup

Want a new way to enjoy broccoli? Where many cream soups can fall short on flavor, this recipe does not. Hot pepper sauce adds a kick of flavor to this classic soup and will surely warm up your taste buds.

MAKES 4 SERVINGS

INGREDIENTS

- 1 cup low sodium vegetable broth
- 3 cups low fat milk
- 1 ½ pounds fresh broccoli, finely chopped
- 2 tablespoons plain nonfat yogurt
- 1 clove garlic, finely chopped
- ⅛ teaspoon ground nutmeg
- ¼ teaspoon onion powder
- ¼ teaspoon hot pepper sauce
- 2 tablespoons all-purpose flour

INSTRUCTIONS

1. In a large soup pot, combine vegetable broth, milk, and broccoli and bring to a boil. Lower heat, cover and simmer for 10 minutes.
2. Add yogurt, garlic, nutmeg, onion powder, and hot pepper sauce. Stir well.
3. Mix in flour and stir until thickened.
4. Heat through and serve.

Mexican Squash Soup

If you like a little heat in your meals, you will love this dish. The slightly sweet butternut squash gets a spicy kick with cumin and chili powder. The brown rice adds nice texture and makes this spicy soup a filling feast!

MAKES 6 SERVINGS

INGREDIENTS

- 1 butternut squash, peeled, cut in half and seeded
- 1 small onion, diced
- 2 cloves garlic, chopped
- 1 tablespoon olive oil
- 4 cups low sodium vegetable broth
- 1 medium tomato, chopped
- ½ cup corn niblets
- ½ teaspoon ground cumin
- ¼ teaspoon chili powder
- ¼ teaspoon salt
- ½ teaspoon black pepper
- ½ cup cooked brown rice
- Chopped fresh cilantro, for garnish
- Chopped fresh parsley, for garnish

INSTRUCTIONS

1. Bake butternut squash for 30 minutes. Set aside.
2. In a soup pot, sauté onion and garlic in olive oil for approximately 6 minutes.
3. Add butternut squash and vegetable broth. Bring to a boil and stir until a smooth consistency, approximately 15 minutes.
4. Add tomato, corn, cumin, chili powder, salt, and black pepper. Cover and cook on medium heat for 8-10 minutes.
5. Add brown rice and mix well.
6. Garnish with cilantro and parsley.

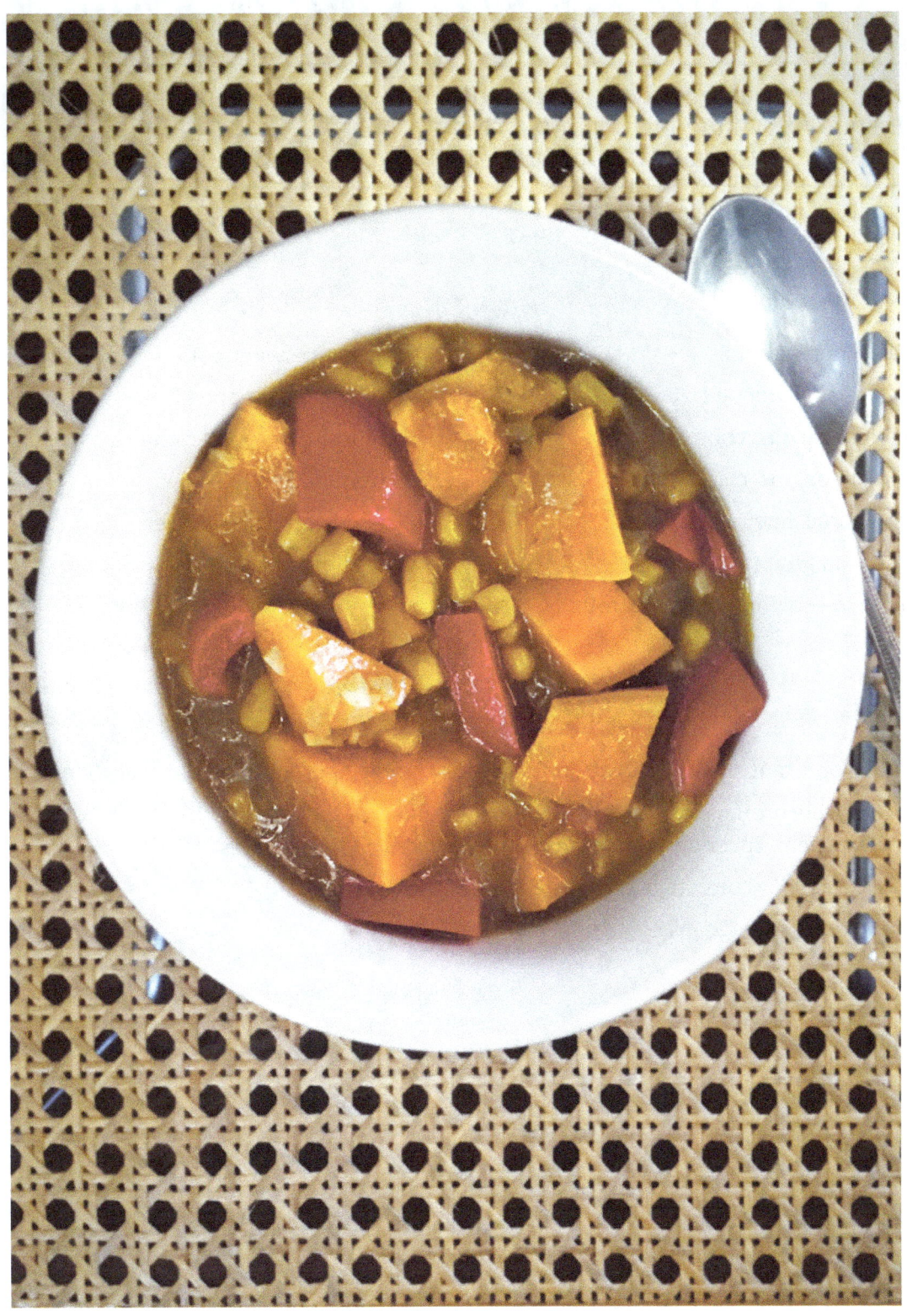

Creamy Sweet Potato Soup

This soup is called creamy for a reason! With warming seasonings like cinnamon and ginger, everything blends into a creamy, hearty sweet potato bliss. Make this for your family on a cool night to warm you up.

MAKES 15 SERVINGS

INGREDIENTS

- 1 tablespoon olive oil
- 1 stalk celery, chopped
- 2 medium carrots, chopped
- 2 medium onions, chopped
- 1 clove garlic, finely chopped
- ⅛ teaspoon ground ginger
- 8 cups low sodium vegetable broth
- 6 medium sweet potatoes, peeled and cubed
- ½ teaspoon chopped fresh thyme
- ½ teaspoon ground cinnamon
- ½ teaspoon salt
- ¼ teaspoon black pepper
- Splash of orange juice

INSTRUCTIONS

1. In a soup pot, sauté celery, carrots, onions, garlic, and ginger for approximately 5 minutes.
2. Add vegetable broth, sweet potatoes, thyme, cinnamon, salt, and black pepper. Bring to a boil then lower heat, cover and simmer for approximately 50-55 minutes.
3. Blend to a chunky consistency or puree if preferred.
4. Add a splash of orange juice and heat through.

Onion Soup

This soup is soup-er savory thanks to the addition of soy sauce and dry mustard. With onion and garlic taking center stage, this soup is packed with vitamin C, flavonoids, and phytonutrients.

MAKES 8 SERVINGS

INGREDIENTS

- 4 large onions, thinly sliced
- 2 cloves garlic, crushed
- 1 tablespoon olive oil
- ½ teaspoon dry mustard
- ⅛ teaspoon thyme
- 1 ½ quart low sodium vegetable broth
- ½ teaspoon onion flakes
- ½ teaspoon onion powder
- 1 tablespoon low sodium soy sauce
- 3 tablespoons dry white wine
- ⅛ teaspoon white pepper

INSTRUCTIONS

1. In a soup pot, sauté the onions and garlic in olive oil until very brown.
2. Add dry mustard and thyme. Mix well.
3. Add vegetable broth and remaining ingredients. Bring to a boil, then lower heat and cook for 30-40 minutes.

Mushroom Barley Soup

It's hard to believe such a hearty tasting soup is completely vegetarian! The mushrooms in this soup absorb the wonderful flavors of barley and onion while adding nice texture. You will savor every last drop.

MAKES 8 SERVINGS

INGREDIENTS

- 1 plum tomato, chopped
- 2 stalks celery, chopped
- 1 medium onion, chopped
- 2 medium carrots, shredded
- 2 cloves garlic, chopped
- 6 cups water
- ½ cup uncooked pearl barley
- ½ cup chopped fresh parsley
- 1 teaspoon salt
- ¼ teaspoon black pepper
- ¼ teaspoon low sodium soy sauce
- 4 cups sliced fresh mushrooms

INSTRUCTIONS

1. In a large soup pot, combine tomato, celery, onion, carrots, and garlic. Add water and bring to a boil.
2. Lower heat. Mix in barley, parsley, salt, black pepper, and soy sauce. Cover and simmer for 45-55 minutes.
3. Add mushrooms and continue to cook for an additional 15 minutes.

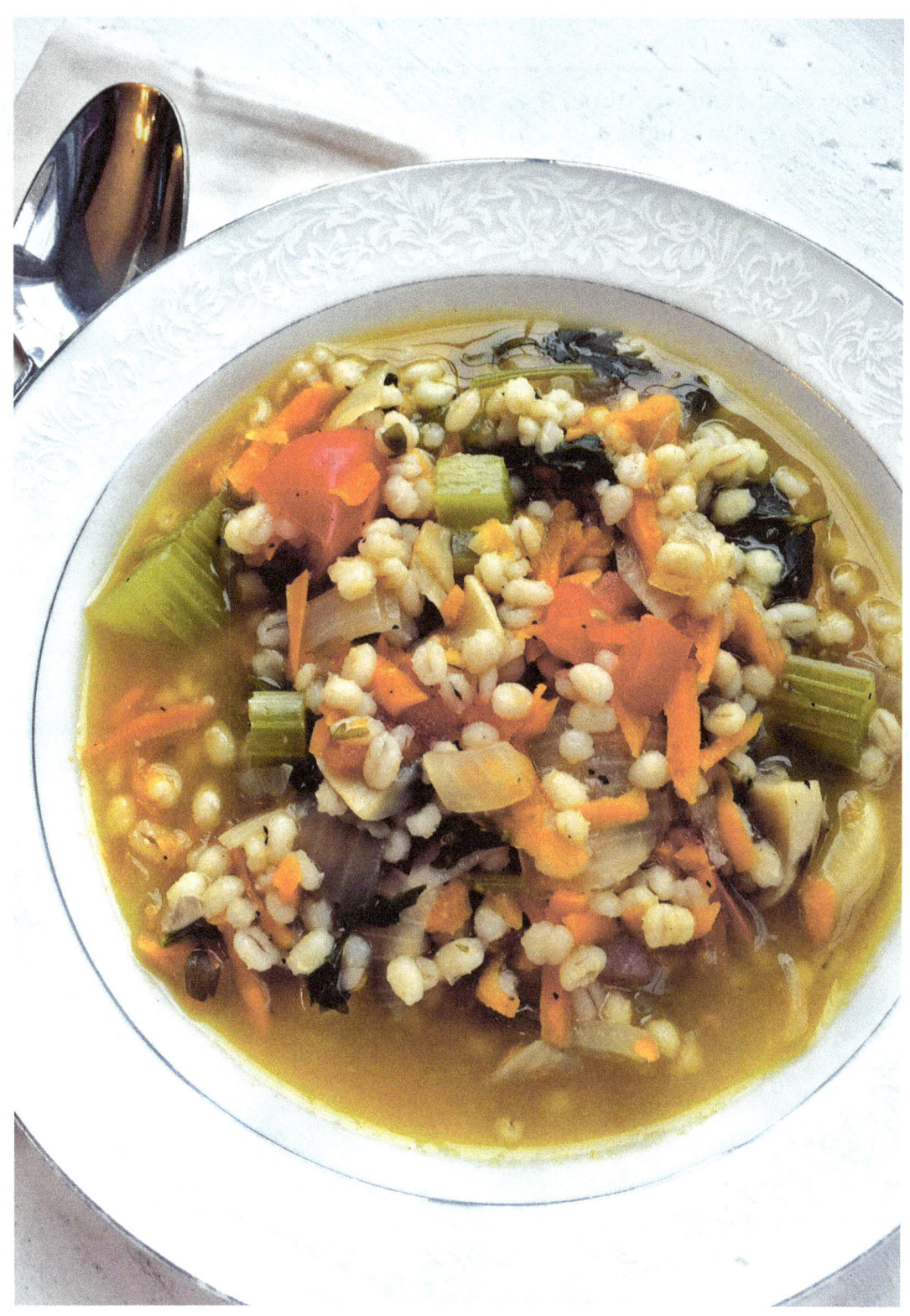

Corn Chowder

As delicious as chowders can be, their creaminess often can be heavy. Not in this chowder! This recipe is light and delivers the creaminess you crave along with the naturally sweet flavor of corn.

MAKES 5 SERVINGS

INGREDIENTS

- 1 tablespoon butter
- 1 medium onion, sliced
- 2 tablespoons all-purpose flour
- 4 cups low fat milk
- 1 teaspoon salt
- 2 cups frozen or canned corn niblets

INSTRUCTIONS

1. In a soup pot, melt margarine and brown onions.
2. Remove pot from flame and stir in flour to coat onions.
3. Return to medium flame and add milk, salt, and corn.
4. Heat until milk is hot, but not boiling, and soup is of a thickened consistency, approximately 30 minutes.

Pasta Fagioli Soup

Who knew one soup could contain so many tasty ingredients? Packed with veggies, mushrooms, kidney beans, pasta, and more, there is something in it for everybody to enjoy. This soup is hearty, filling, and will easily become a favorite.

MAKES 12 SERVINGS

INGREDIENTS

- 3 ½ cups low sodium vegetable broth, divided
- ½ cup white wine
- 1 clove garlic, minced
- 1 small onion, diced
- 1 small green bell pepper, diced
- 1 medium carrot, diced
- 2 stalks celery, diced
- ½ teaspoon dried thyme
- 2 plum tomatoes, diced
- 6 fresh mushrooms, quartered
- 1 small eggplant, diced
- 2 tablespoons tomato paste
- 1 (10-ounce) can kidney beans, drained and rinsed
- 1 teaspoon dried oregano
- 1 bay leaf
- 1 cup uncooked ditalini pasta

INSTRUCTIONS

1. In a soup pot, bring ½ cup vegetable broth and wine to a simmer.
2. Add garlic, onion, green pepper, carrot, celery, and thyme. Simmer for 4-5 minutes.
3. Add tomatoes, mushrooms, eggplant, tomato paste, beans, oregano, and bay leaf.
4. Add remaining 3 cups of vegetable broth and pasta. Cook until pasta is tender, approximately 25-30 minutes. If needed, add water or broth to achieve desired consistency.

Creamy Tomato Soup

with Couscous

Flavors of the Mediterranean are certainly delivered in this soup. Cilantro and cumin will tingle your tongue, while the couscous is a fun addition. This soup will take you on a flavor vacation to the Mediterranean.

MAKES 10 SERVINGS

INGREDIENTS

- 1 medium onion, chopped
- 2 medium carrots, diced
- 1 tablespoon olive oil
- 1 (14 ½ -ounce) can crushed tomatoes
- 6 cloves garlic, chopped
- 4 cups low sodium vegetable broth
- 3 cups plain soy milk
- ¼ teaspoon ground cumin
- ¼ bunch fresh cilantro, chopped
- Cayenne pepper, to taste
- Black pepper, to taste
- 4-ounces uncooked couscous

INSTRUCTIONS

1. In a soup pot, sauté onion and carrots in olive oil for approximately 10 minutes.
2. Add the tomatoes, garlic, vegetable broth, soy milk, cumin, cilantro, cayenne pepper, and black pepper.
3. Bring to a boil, then reduce heat and simmer for 10 minutes.
4. Remove from heat and let cool slightly. Using an immersion or free-standing blender, blend until smooth.
5. Add couscous and cook for approximately 10-15 minutes or until the couscous is soft.
6. Serve immediately, otherwise the couscous will absorb the liquid and the dish will become too thick.

Strawberries & Crème Soup

Dessert soups are a delicious way to incorporate fruit in a not-so-typical way. The orange juice adds just the right amount of zing and acidity which compliments the sweet strawberries. The yogurt adds a silky texture to create an unexpected treat.

MAKES 5 SERVINGS

INGREDIENTS

- 1 pound fresh strawberries
- 1 small banana
- ½ cup orange juice
- ½ teaspoon vanilla extract
- 1 tablespoon lemon juice
- 2 cups plain nonfat yogurt
- 1 tablespoon mint, for garnish

INSTRUCTIONS

1. In a blender, combine strawberries, banana, and orange juice.
2. Add vanilla extract, lemon juice, and yogurt.
3. Blend until all the ingredients are combined well.
4. Chill for at least 2 hours.
5. Garnish with mint before serving.

Intuitive Eating Wisdom

In order to make peace with food, you must become a priority in your own life. Taking time to reflect on and honor your body will create space for you to learn to trust your body. It knows what, when, and how much to eat, which will guide you to find peace in your eating.

Salads

IN THIS CHAPTER

- 35 | Colorful Health Salad
- 36 | Black Bean & Wild Rice Romaine Salad
- 38 | Outrageous Caesar Salad
- 39 | Mixed Greens & Mango Salad
- 40 | Cherry Chili Pepper Salad
- 42 | Pickled Green Bean Salad
- 43 | Jicama Salad
- 44 | Marinated Vegetable Medley
- 46 | Italian Herb Tomato Salad
- 47 | Chickpea Salad
- 48 | Mixed Greens Citrus Berry Salad
- 50 | Shredded Carrot & Raisin Salad

Salads

Colorful Health Salad

A lot of color is a sure sign you are getting a variety of powerful nutrients. This is a refreshing and delightful twist to the everyday coleslaw. It will certainly become a fan favorite in your home.

MAKES 6 SERVINGS

SALAD INGREDIENTS

- 1 cup shredded white cabbage
- 1 cup shredded red cabbage
- ½ cup shredded carrots
- ½ cup chopped green bell pepper
- ½ cup chopped red bell pepper
- ¼ cup chopped red onion
- 1 ½ tablespoons minced fresh parsley

DRESSING INGREDIENTS

- ¼ cup vinegar
- ¼ cup light Italian dressing
- 1 ½ teaspoons sugar
- ⅛ teaspoon black pepper

INSTRUCTIONS

1. In a large bowl, combine cabbage, carrots, green and red peppers, red onion, and parsley. Mix well and set aside.
2. Combine vinegar, Italian dressing, sugar, and black pepper in a jar; cover tightly and shake vigorously.
3. Pour dressing mixture over vegetables, tossing gently to coat well.
4. Cover and refrigerate until thoroughly chilled.
5. Stir coleslaw lightly before serving. Serve using a slotted spoon.

Black Bean & Wild Rice Romaine Salad

Rice and beans are a match made in food heaven. Adding them to a classic salad can make any mouth water. This salad is a great entrée packed with fiber, protein and vegetables—everything you want in a wholesome meal!

MAKES 12 SERVINGS

INGREDIENTS

- 1 (16-ounce) can black beans, drained and rinsed, or ⅔ cup dry black beans
- ½ cup uncooked wild rice
- 1 cup chopped red bell pepper
- 1 cucumber, sliced
- ⅛ teaspoon black pepper
- 1 head romaine lettuce, chopped
- 16 ounces feta cheese
- 3 tablespoons slivered almonds
- ¼ cup prepared light raspberry vinaigrette dressing

INSTRUCTIONS

1. If using canned beans, skip ahead. If using dry beans, soak in 3 cups water for up to 8 hours or overnight in the refrigerator. Drain and rinse. Combine beans with 3 cups of fresh water and simmer for 1 ½-2 hours or until tender. Drain.
2. Cook wild rice according to package directions; cool to room temperature.
3. In a large bowl, combine black beans and rice with red pepper, cucumber, black pepper, and romaine lettuce.
4. Sprinkle feta cheese and almonds on top of the salad.
5. Drizzle dressing over salad and toss.

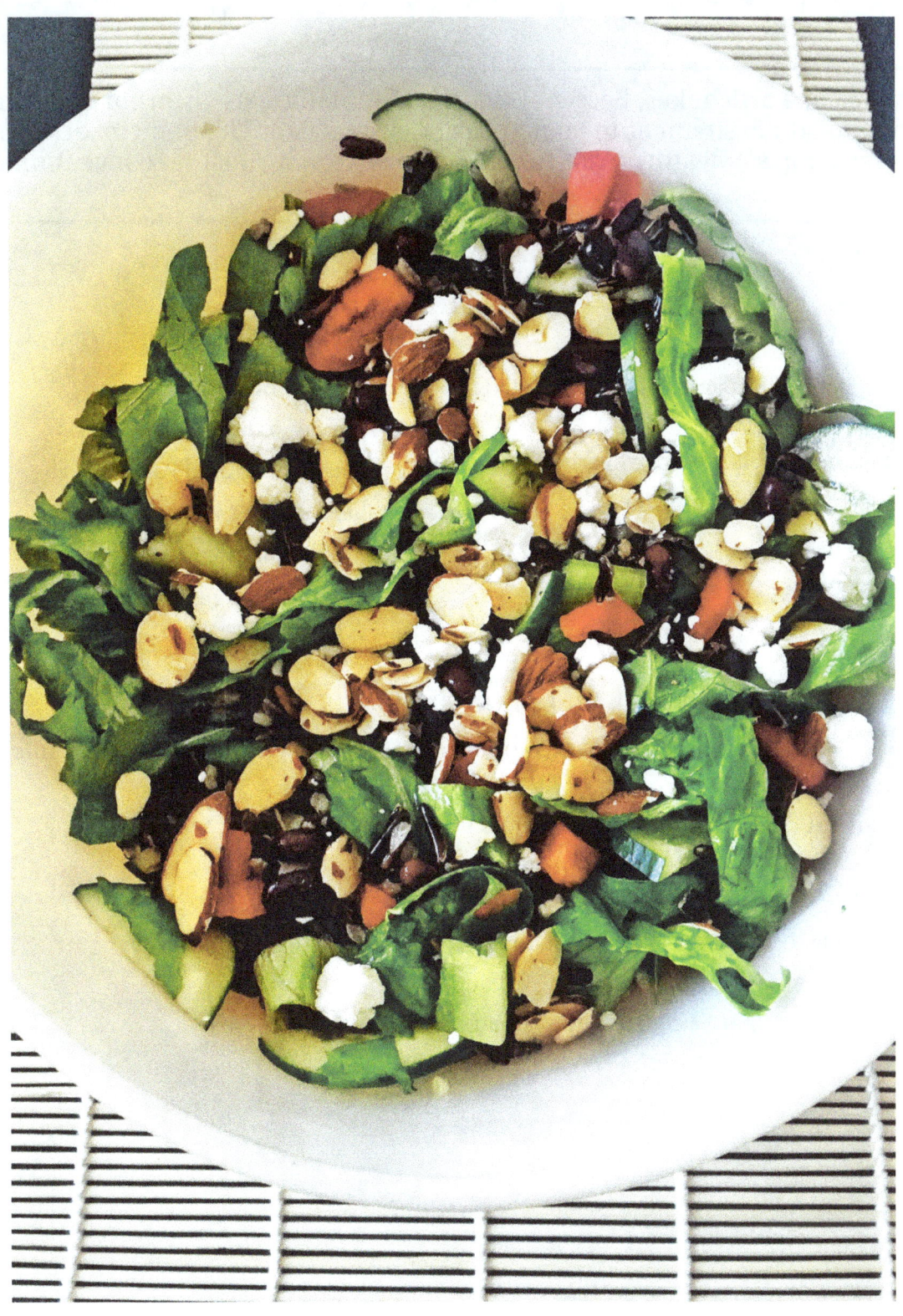

Outrageous Caesar Salad

Vegetables like artichokes, hearts of palm and tomatoes are incorporated into this recipe to add excitement to your typical Caesar salad. The homemade Caesar dressing has a healthy twist to make it stand out against its conventional counterpart.

MAKES 10 SERVINGS

SALAD INGREDIENTS

- 1 medium head romaine lettuce, torn into bite-size pieces
- 1 ½ cups quartered artichoke hearts
- 1 ½ cups sliced hearts of palm
- 1 ½ cups halved cherry tomatoes
- 1 cup croutons

DRESSING INGREDIENTS

- ⅓ cup light sour cream
- 2 tablespoons light mayonnaise
- 2 tablespoons grated Parmesan cheese
- 1 tablespoon red wine vinegar
- 1 teaspoon minced garlic
- ⅛ teaspoon black pepper

INSTRUCTIONS

1. In large bowl, mix lettuce, artichoke hearts, hearts of palm, cherry tomatoes, and croutons. Set aside.
2. Combine sour cream, mayonnaise, Parmesan cheese, vinegar, garlic, and black pepper. Blend well.
3. Refrigerate dressing several hours.
4. When ready to serve, toss salad with dressing and serve.

For an alternative Caesar Salad Dressing see page 59.

Mixed Greens & Mango Salad

Three words describe this recipe: colorful, delicious, and nutritious! The avocado provides a creamy texture and the craisins, mango, and orange add sweetness and color to this delicious dish. Highlighting not-so-common salad ingredients, this dish will be a hit at any get-together.

MAKES 10 SERVINGS

SALAD INGREDIENTS

- 4 cups mixed greens
- 1 small red onion, thinly sliced
- 1 small mango, cut into chunks
- 1 medium orange, peeled and segmented
- 1 avocado, diced
- 2 tablespoons craisins

DRESSING INGREDIENTS

- ¼ cup white wine vinegar
- 1 teaspoon Dijon mustard
- 2 tablespoons olive oil

INSTRUCTIONS

1. In a large bowl, mix greens, red onion, mango, and orange.
2. In a separate bowl, whisk together white wine vinegar, Dijon mustard, and olive oil. Pour over salad and toss well.
3. Top salad with avocado and craisins.

Cherry Chili Pepper Salad

Opposites attract when tart cherries are mixed with spicy chili pepper. This unique salad has a lovely variety of vegetables to balance out these two dominant flavors. Its bright colors and flavors make this salad a perfect addition to the table.

MAKES 7 SERVINGS

SALAD INGREDIENTS

- 1¼ cups pitted fresh sweet cherries
- 1 cup thinly sliced green bell pepper
- 1 cup thinly sliced red bell pepper
- ¼ cup finely chopped chili pepper, seeds removed
- 2 tablespoons finely chopped onion
- 4 cups mixed greens

DRESSING INGREDIENTS

- 2 tablespoons white wine vinegar
- ½ tablespoon olive oil
- 2 teaspoons sugar
- ⅛ teaspoon salt
- ⅛ teaspoon black pepper

INSTRUCTIONS

1. In a large bowl, toss together cherries, green and red peppers, chili pepper, and onions.
2. In a separate bowl, mix white wine vinegar, olive oil, sugar, salt, and black pepper. Pour over cherry and pepper mixture and toss well.
3. Serve over mixed greens.

Salads

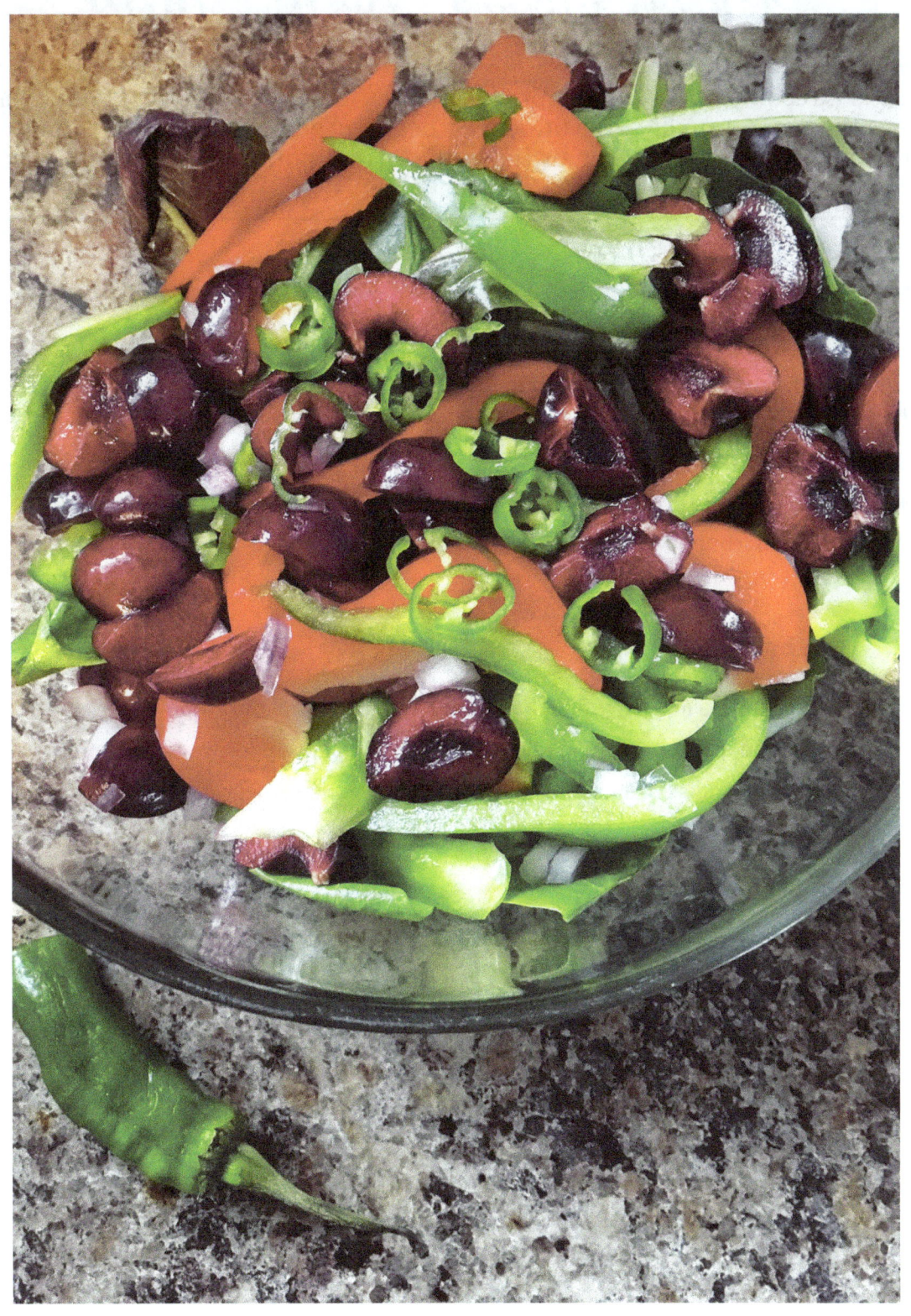

Pickled Green Bean Salad

This is a recipe that should be prepared days in advance so the green beans achieve the perfect pickled flavor. Green beans provide fiber and vitamin C and pair wonderfully with chicken or fish and roasted potatoes for a well-balanced meal.

MAKES 4 SERVINGS

INGREDIENTS

- 8-ounces fresh French green beans, trimmed and rinsed
- 2 tablespoons red wine vinegar
- 1 teaspoon sugar
- ½ small red onion, chopped
- 2 tablespoons minced fresh dill
- ⅛ teaspoon salt
- ⅛ teaspoon black pepper
- 1 cup water

INSTRUCTIONS

1. Place beans lengthwise in a jar with tight-fitting lid. Beans should fit somewhat tight in jar.
2. Pour in vinegar and add sugar, onion, dill, salt, and black pepper.
3. Add water to fill jar and seal. Shake to blend ingredients and refrigerate for three days before serving.

Salads

Jicama Salad

This salad has cool, refreshing flavors with a dressing that packs a punch! Give jicama a try in this twist on a classic cucumber salad. It's a healthy side for a summer BBQ or a tangy start to any meal.

MAKES 7 SERVINGS

SALAD INGREDIENTS

- 1 (8-ounce) jicama, peeled and cut into ½-inch sticks
- 1 small cucumber, thinly sliced
- 1 medium orange, peeled and segmented

DRESSING INGREDIENTS

- ¼ cup white wine vinegar
- 2 tablespoons olive oil
- 1 teaspoon fresh lemon juice
- ¼ teaspoon chili powder
- ¼ teaspoon salt

INSTRUCTIONS

1. In a serving bowl, combine jicama, cucumber, and orange segments.
2. In a separate bowl, whisk together vinegar, oil, lemon juice, chili powder, and salt. Pour over the jicama mixture and toss well.
3. Chill in the refrigerator overnight.

Marinated Vegetable Medley

This salad is the epitome of eating the colors of the rainbow. You will be treating yourself to an abundance of flavors and powerful nutrients!

MAKES 12 SERVINGS

SALAD INGREDIENTS

- 1 (14-ounce) can artichoke hearts, drained and rinsed
- 1 cucumber, chopped
- 1 red bell pepper, chopped
- 1 medium head cauliflower, chopped
- 1 medium head fresh broccoli, chopped
- 1 small onion, diced
- ½ cup green beans, cut into ½-inch pieces
- 1 medium tomato, chopped

DRESSING INGREDIENTS

- ½ cup apple cider vinegar
- 2 tablespoons lemon juice
- 2 teaspoons olive oil
- 2 cloves garlic, chopped
- 2 tablespoons chopped fresh parsley
- 2 teaspoons oregano

INSTRUCTIONS

1. In a large bowl, combine artichoke hearts, cucumber, red pepper, cauliflower, broccoli, onion, green beans, and tomato.
2. In a separate bowl, whisk together apple cider vinegar, lemon juice, olive oil, garlic, parsley, and oregano. Pour over vegetables.
3. Chill for at least 12 hours.

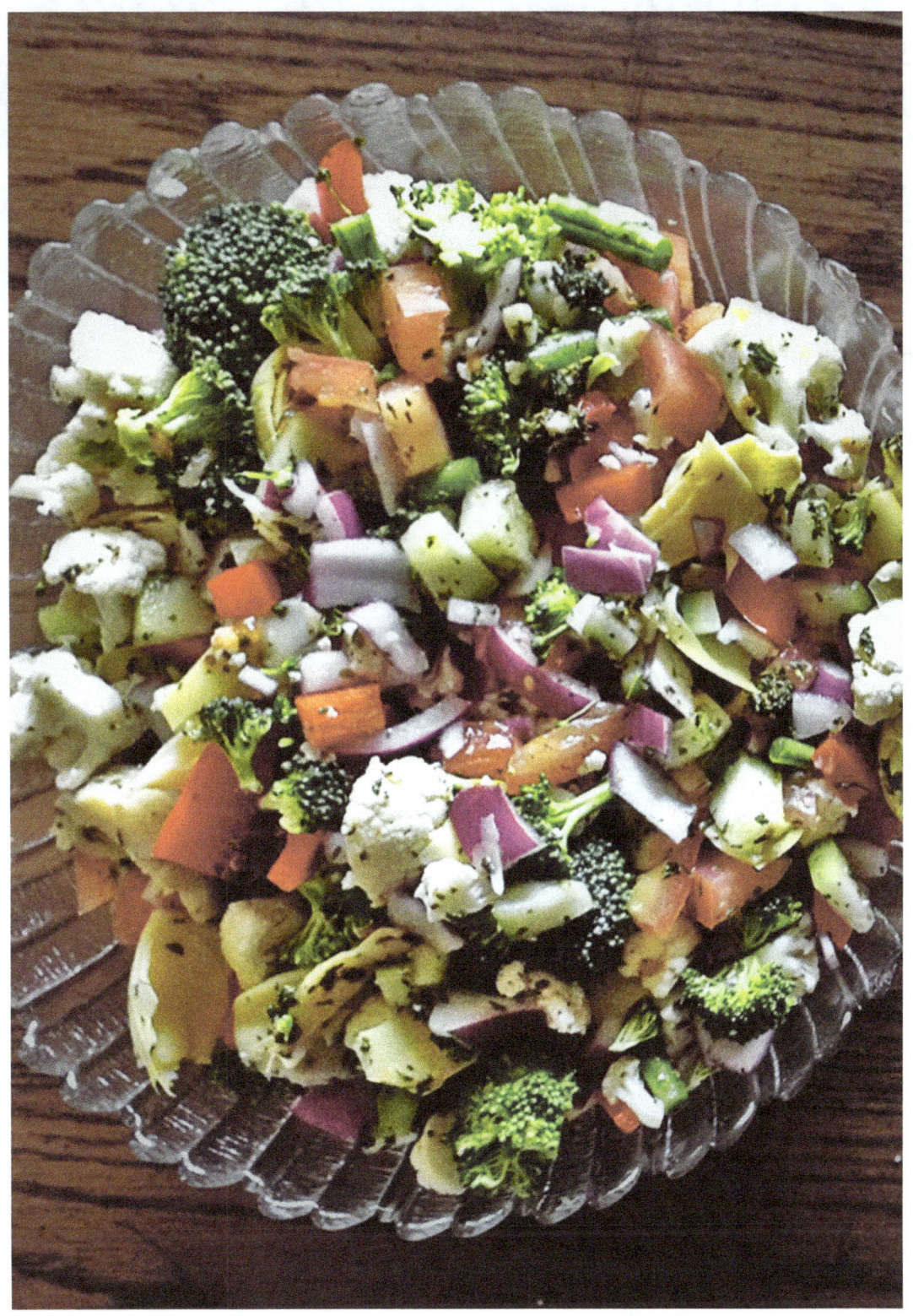

Italian Herb Tomato Salad

Tomatoes are often a side-kick in a salad, but in this dish they take a starring role. The aromatic herbs will remind you of your favorite tomato sauce, but in salad form!

MAKES 4 SERVINGS

INGREDIENTS

- 2 large tomatoes, sliced
- ¼ cup red wine vinegar
- ¼ teaspoon Italian herb seasoning
- ⅛ teaspoon black pepper
- ⅛ teaspoon garlic powder

INSTRUCTIONS

1. Arrange tomatoes in a shallow bowl.
2. In a separate bowl, mix vinegar, Italian herb seasoning, black pepper, and garlic powder. Pour over tomatoes.
3. Let tomatoes marinate for 30 minutes to 4 hours before serving.

Chickpea Salad

There are many versions of the chickpea salad found in supermarkets and delis that are packed with oil and sodium. Why not make your own? The healthy dressing and vibrant veggies in this salad will make this version stand out over store-bought salads any day.

MAKES 6 SERVINGS

SALAD INGREDIENTS

- 1 (15-ounce) can chickpeas, drained and rinsed
- 5 artichoke hearts, chopped
- 1 cup halved cherry tomatoes
- ½ cup halved green olives
- ½ cup diced orange bell pepper
- ½ cup diced yellow bell pepper
- ⅓ cup sliced scallions
- 1 tablespoon chopped fresh parsley

DRESSING INGREDIENTS

- 1 tablespoon olive oil
- 1 ½ tablespoon apple cider vinegar
- 1 clove garlic, minced

INSTRUCTIONS

1. In a large mixing bowl, combine chickpeas, artichokes, cherry tomatoes, olives, bell peppers, scallions, and parsley.
2. In a separate bowl, whisk together olive oil, apple cider vinegar, and garlic.
3. Toss salad with dressing. Refrigerate until chilled.

Mixed Greens Citrus Berry Salad

Berries bursting with sweetness, crunchy walnuts, and a bed of mixed greens results in a zesty, texture party for your taste buds. This is the perfect way to incorporate fruit into your dinner.

MAKES 6 SERVINGS

SALAD INGREDIENTS

- 5 cups mixed greens
- ½ cup fresh blueberries
- ½ cup quartered fresh strawberries
- 1 medium orange, peeled, segmented, and cut into chunks
- ⅛ cup chopped walnuts

DRESSING INGREDIENTS

- 2 tablespoons olive oil
- ¼ cup apple cider vinegar
- 2 tablespoons light brown sugar

INSTRUCTIONS

1. In a large bowl, mix together greens, blueberries, strawberries, oranges, and walnuts.
2. In a jar, combine olive oil, apple cider vinegar, and brown sugar and shake well. Pour over salad and toss well.
3. Chill in refrigerator for at least 1 hour before serving.

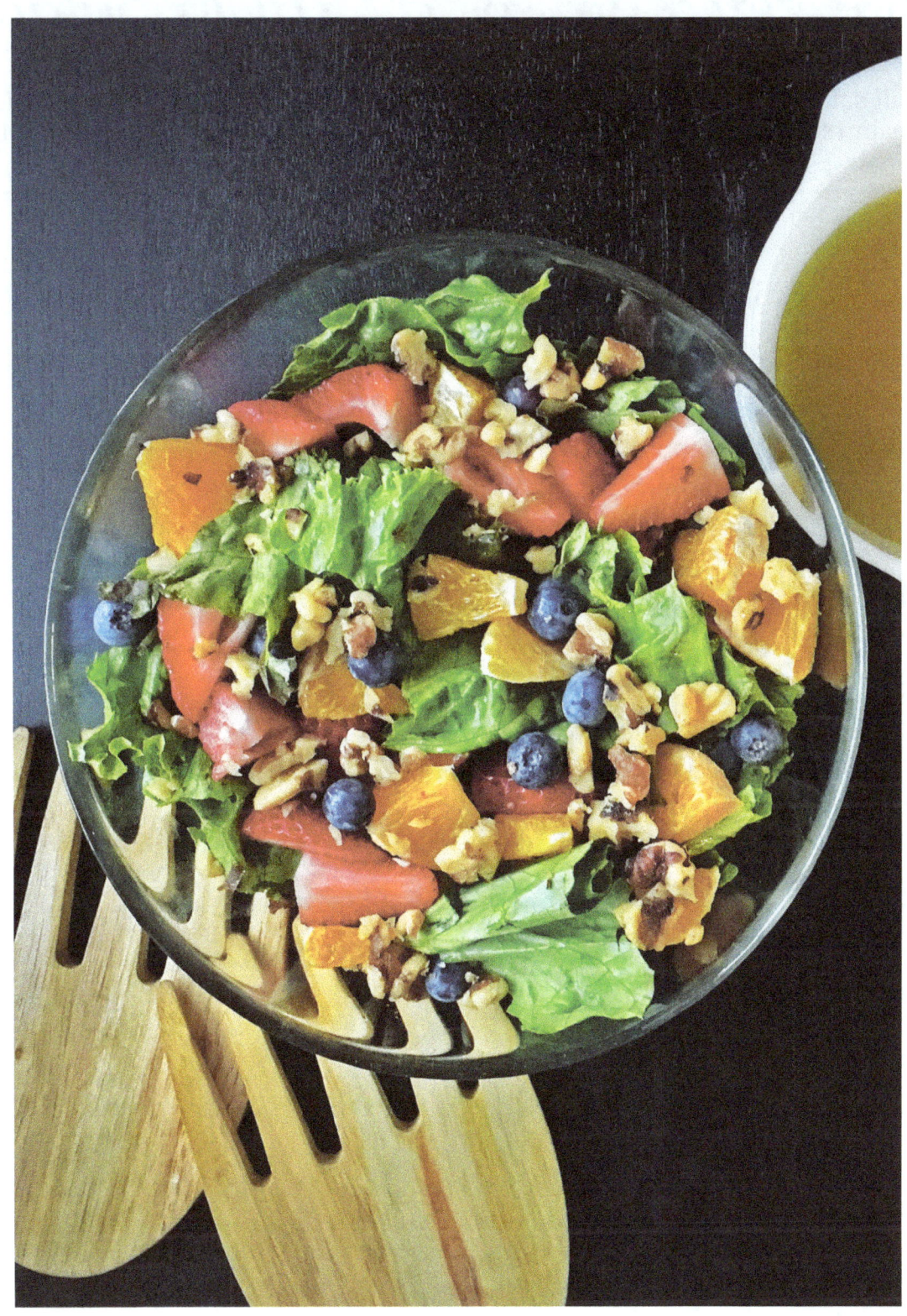

Shredded Carrot & Raisin Salad

Not all salads need lettuce! This is a carrot-based salad with apples and raisins that is bursting with sweet flavors. The creamy dressing gives a refreshing taste and smooth texture to the crunchy carrots.

MAKES 6 SERVINGS

SALAD INGREDIENTS

- 1 pound carrots, peeled and shredded
- 1 ½ cups shredded apples
- ¼ cup dark raisins

DRESSING INGREDIENTS

- ½ cup plain nonfat yogurt
- ⅓ cup low fat milk
- 1 tablespoon lemon juice
- 3 tablespoons sugar
- ¼ teaspoon ground nutmeg
- ¼ teaspoon ground cinnamon

INSTRUCTIONS

1. In a large bowl, combine carrots, apples, and raisins.
2. In a separate bowl, combine yogurt, milk, lemon juice, sugar, nutmeg, and cinnamon. Mix well and spoon over carrot mixture. Toss to coat.
3. Refrigerate and serve chilled.

Intuitive Eating Wisdom

Food provides the fuel for your body. You CAN take charge of your nutrition decisions to support a healthy body and life. This means taking a step back from the restrictions of dieting and opening your mind to eating foods that suit your needs and desires.

Dips & Dressings

IN THIS CHAPTER
---

55 | Classic Marinade

56 | Yogurt Dill Sauce

58 | Balsamic Vinaigrette

59 | Caesar Dressing

60 | Spinach Artichoke Dip

62 | Honey Mustard Dressing

63 | Tofu-Avocado Dip

64 | Pineapple Salsa

66 | Hummus

67 | Spicy Salsa

Dips & Dressings

Classic Marinade

Experience the subtle hint of herbs in this quick and easy marinade. Great for use before or during cooking to add a savory flavor to your meat, poultry, fish, and veggies.

MAKES 5 SERVINGS

INGREDIENTS

- ½ cup white wine vinegar
- 1 tablespoon olive oil
- ¼ cup finely chopped onion
- 1 small bay leaf
- ½ teaspoon dried rosemary
- 2 cloves garlic, finely minced
- ½ teaspoon black pepper

INSTRUCTIONS

1. In a medium bowl, combine all ingredients until well blended.
2. Add food to be marinated and turn several times until all sides are coated.
3. Cover and refrigerate for at least 30 minutes, occasionally turning food so that marinade is evenly distributed.

Yogurt Dill Sauce

This recipe is a multipurpose spread! Its light and creamy flavor is perfect for sandwiches and works great as a dip or sauce. Drizzle on baked chicken, use it as a dip for baby carrots, or spread it on a turkey sandwich. The possibilities are endless!

MAKES 4 SERVINGS

INGREDIENTS

- ¼ cup plain nonfat yogurt
- ¼ cup light mayonnaise
- 2 tablespoons chopped dill
- ¼ teaspoon salt

INSTRUCTIONS

1. In a small bowl, mix all ingredients together.
2. Cover and refrigerate until ready to serve.

Dips & Dressings

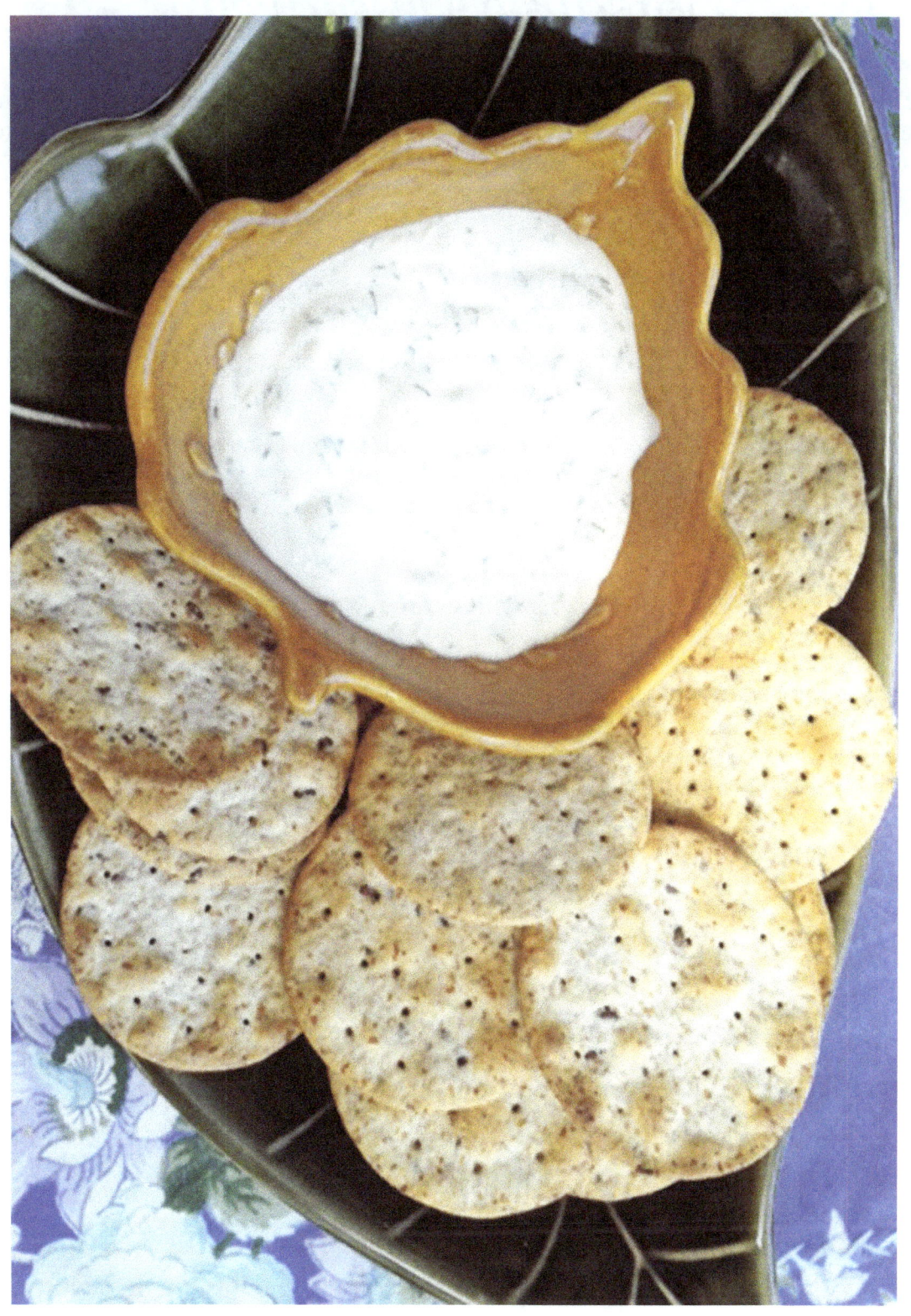

Balsamic Vinaigrette

Utilizing common kitchen ingredients, this popular dressing is easy to whip up at home. Have it handy in your refrigerator to toss on top of salads, grilled chicken, or fresh tomatoes and mozzarella.

MAKES 5 SERVINGS

INGREDIENTS

- ⅓ cup balsamic vinegar
- 2 tablespoons olive oil
- 2 tablespoons water
- 1 teaspoon sugar
- ¼ teaspoon salt
- ⅛ teaspoon black pepper
- 1 teaspoon Dijon mustard
- ½ clove garlic, crushed

INSTRUCTIONS

1. Combine all ingredients and mix well.
2. Cover and refrigerate until ready to serve.

Dips & Dressings

Caesar Dressing

Caesar dressing is a popular option for both restaurants and home-cooking. With this recipe, you can make your own version at home while still enjoying the same creamy, flavorful dressing you would get from the bottle.

MAKES 6 SERVINGS

INGREDIENTS

- ¼ cup lemon juice
- ¼ cup cider vinegar
- ¼ cup water
- 3 tablespoons grated Parmesan cheese
- 2 tablespoons Dijon mustard
- 1 teaspoon garlic powder
- 1 teaspoon black pepper

INSTRUCTIONS

1. In a small bowl, mix all ingredients together.
2. Cover and store in refrigerator until ready to serve.

Spinach Artichoke Dip

Impress your guests with this dip that seems fancy, but is easy to make! Serve this creamy, appetizing dip with whole grain crackers or veggies at your next get-together or with your mid-day snack.

MAKES 26 SERVINGS

INGREDIENTS

- 2 cups plain nonfat yogurt
- ½ cup light mayonnaise
- 1 teaspoon salt
- 1 teaspoon sugar
- 2 scallions, chopped
- 1 (10-ounce) box frozen spinach, thawed and strained
- 1 (14-ounce) jar artichoke hearts, chopped

INSTRUCTIONS

1. In a medium bowl, combine yogurt, mayonnaise, salt, and sugar.
2. Add scallions, spinach, and artichokes and mix well.
3. Serve with vegetables, crackers, or spoon into a hollowed-out loaf of bread and serve with bite-size pieces of bread.

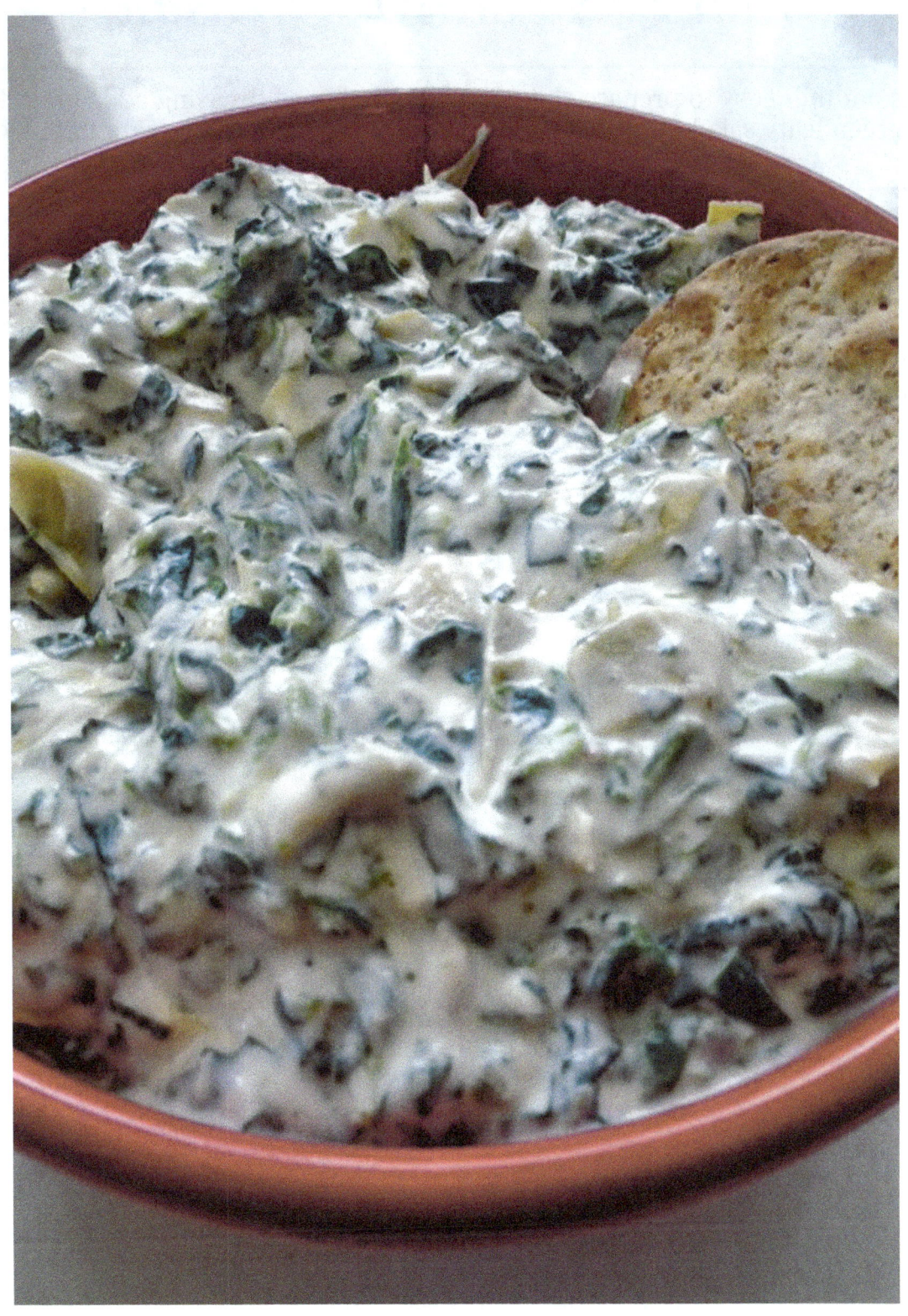

Honey Mustard Dressing

This is another easy to prepare classic. Honey mustard dressing adds great flavor to a green leafy salad but is also a tasty choice for a slightly sweet marinade for meat or poultry.

MAKES 12 SERVINGS

INGREDIENTS

- ¼ cup sugar
- ¼ cup honey
- ¼ cup white wine vinegar
- 1 tablespoon Dijon mustard
- ½ cup water
- ⅛ cup olive oil
- ¼ cup chopped onion

INSTRUCTIONS

1. Combine all ingredients and mix well.
2. Cover and refrigerate until ready to serve.

Tofu-Avocado Dip

This tofu and avocado mixture is packed with protein and healthy fats and is a twist on regular guacamole. It's a great addition to any fiesta!

MAKES 8 SERVINGS

INGREDIENTS

- 1 (6-ounce) block soft tofu, drained
- 1 medium avocado, peeled and mashed
- 2 tablespoons low fat sour cream
- ½ teaspoon salt
- 1 tablespoon lemon juice
- ¼ cup finely chopped onion
- 4 drops hot sauce
- ⅛ teaspoon black pepper
- 1 tablespoon finely chopped fresh parsley

INSTRUCTIONS

1. Place all ingredients in a blender and puree 30 seconds or until smooth consistency.
2. Cover and refrigerate for 1 hour or until ready to serve.
3. Serve with raw vegetables, as a salad dressing, mixed with tuna, or as a topping for baked potatoes.

Pineapple Salsa

This salsa recipe has a sweet flavor with a spicy punch that can turn a bland dish into a flavorful one in no time. Easy to make and delicious in taste, this is sure to be a family favorite. It's a great addition to grilled or broiled fish.

MAKES 5 SERVINGS

INGREDIENTS

- 1 cup finely chopped fresh pineapple
- 1 tablespoon finely chopped red onion
- 1 tablespoon finely chopped scallions
- 2 tablespoons finely chopped red bell pepper
- 1 tablespoon finely chopped fresh cilantro
- 1 tablespoon honey
- ⅛ teaspoon ground red pepper
- 1 ½ tablespoons lime juice
- ¼ teaspoon black pepper
- 2 teaspoons minced jalapeno pepper (optional)

INSTRUCTIONS

1. Combine all ingredients.
2. Cover and refrigerate for an hour or more to blend flavors.

Dips & Dressings

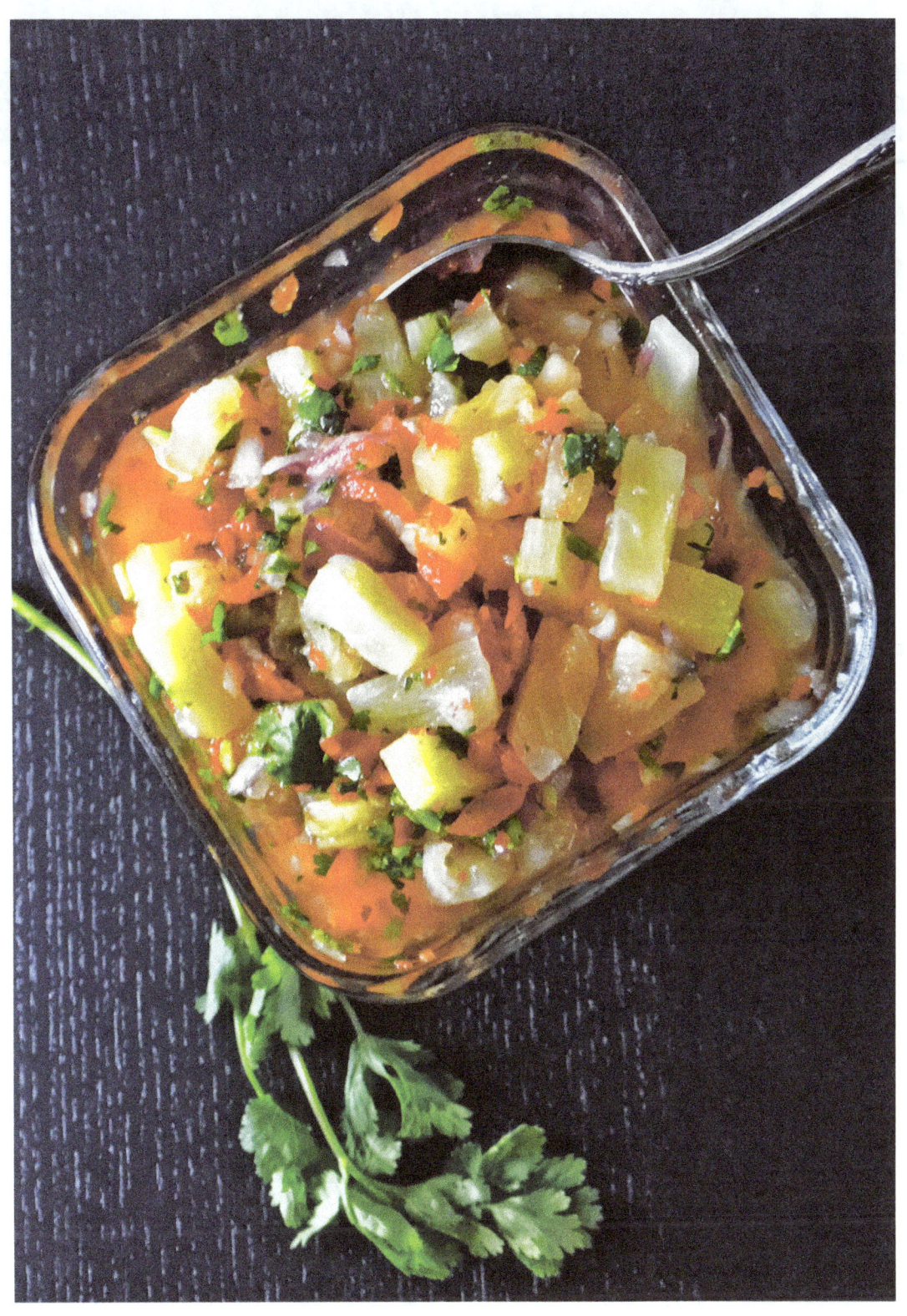

Hummus

Hummus is a popular protein-packed staple used for dipping veggies and crackers. Use this quick and easy recipe to make your own homemade classic style hummus!

MAKES 24 SERVINGS

INGREDIENTS

- 2 (15-ounce) cans chickpeas, drained and rinsed
- 2 tablespoons tahini
- Juice of half a lemon
- 1 teaspoon ground cumin
- 3 cloves garlic
- ½ teaspoon salt
- ¼ teaspoon red cayenne pepper
- ¼ cup boiling water

INSTRUCTIONS

1. Place all ingredients, except boiling water, in a food processor.
2. Slowly add boiling water, blending until smooth consistency. If mixture is too dry and difficult to blend, add more boiling water one tablespoon at a time.
3. Refrigerate for 1 hour or until ready to serve.

Spicy Salsa

Why purchase jarred salsa when you can make your own with this easy but flavorful recipe? With spicy jalapenos and red wine vinegar providing more than a kick of flavor, your guests will cha-cha-cha right to this dip! Serve as a condiment to fish, chicken, or lean beef.

MAKES 6 SERVINGS

INGREDIENTS

- 6 small tomatoes, peeled, seeded, and chopped
- ¾ cup diced red onion
- 3 jalapeno peppers, seeded and diced
- ¼ cup minced fresh cilantro
- ½ cup minced fresh parsley
- 3 cloves garlic, minced
- 3 tablespoons red wine vinegar

INSTRUCTIONS

1. In a medium bowl, combine all ingredients.
2. Cover and refrigerate for at least 1 hour prior to serving.

Intuitive Eating Wisdom

Intuitive Eating Principle 1: Reject the Diet Mentality

It's time to say goodbye for good to the diets and misinformation which promise to shed the pounds. The diet mentality fosters unhealthy restrictive behavior and causes self-doubt and frustration as the weight comes and goes as quickly as the diet does. Shifting out of the diet mentality requires a whole new way of thinking about food and your body. Intuitive eating starts in the mind.

Hot Sides

IN THIS CHAPTER

73 | Very Moist Stuffing

74 | Sautéed Spinach & Leeks

75 | Garden Vegetable Packet

76 | Crunchy Brussels Sprouts

78 | Roasted Vegetable Salad with Basil Vinaigrette

79 | Broccoli Soufflé

80 | Asparagus with Mustard Vinaigrette

82 | Stuffed Grape Leaves

83 | Raisin & Craisin Potato Mounds

84 | Portobello Mushroom Sauté

86 | Baked Sweet Potato Fries

87 | Stuffed Potato Skins

88 | Mock Stuffed Derma

90 | Vibrant Mashed Potatoes

91 | Brown Rice Bake

Hot Sides

IN THIS CHAPTER

92 | Ginger Caraway Carrots

94 | Couscous Salad with Tomatoes & Roasted Red Pepper

95 | Spanish Rice

96 | Penne Pasta with Spinach & Red Kidney Beans

98 | Barley Vegetable Medley

99 | Curried Brown Rice Salad with Green Beans

100 | Tomato Mushroom Barley Risotto

Hot Sides

Very Moist Stuffing

Nothing is worse than dry stuffing. This recipe will ensure that your stuffing will come out moist and flavorful every time. It's so tasty and easy to make that you'll always offer to bring the stuffing for the holidays!

MAKES 8 SERVINGS

INGREDIENTS

- 2 cups diced onions
- 2 cups diced celery
- 2 cups low sodium chicken broth
- ½ tablespoon onion powder
- ½ tablespoon garlic powder
- ½ teaspoon dried parsley
- 1 loaf stuffing bread (approximately 8 cups cubed bread, firm texture)

INSTRUCTIONS

1. Preheat oven to 350°F.
2. In a sauce pan, combine onions, celery, chicken broth, onion powder, garlic powder, and dried parsley.
3. Simmer for 20 minutes or until the vegetables are tender and liquid is reduced by half.
4. Place cubes of bread in a large bowl. Pour onion mixture over the bread cubes and toss to coat.
5. Transfer to a baking dish and cover with aluminum foil. Bake for 25 minutes.

Sautéed Spinach & Leeks

Leeks are similar to onions, but are not as strong in flavor. They add a nice touch to spinach without overpowering it. The pine nuts add crunch and texture to the soft leafy greens.

MAKES 6 SERVINGS

INGREDIENTS

- 2 cloves garlic, minced
- 1 tablespoon olive oil
- 1 leek, white bottom part only, cleaned and thinly sliced
- 2 pounds fresh baby spinach leaves, cleaned
- ¼ teaspoon ground nutmeg
- Salt, to taste
- Black pepper, to taste
- 4 tablespoons pine nuts

INSTRUCTIONS

1. Sauté garlic in olive oil over medium heat. Add leek and sauté for 5 minutes.
2. Add spinach and cook for 3-5 minutes.
3. Add nutmeg and season with salt and black pepper.
4. Sprinkle with pine nuts.

Hot Sides

Garden Vegetable Packet

Need a new way of preparing your vegetables? Bake them in packets! The flavors stay sealed in the foil and the veggies will cook perfectly every time.

MAKES 12 SERVINGS

INGREDIENTS

- 3 cups fresh broccoli florets
- 2 cups fresh cauliflower florets
- ½ medium red bell pepper, cut into 1 inch pieces
- 1 teaspoon dried basil
- ½ teaspoon salt
- ⅛ teaspoon black pepper
- 2 ice cubes

INSTRUCTIONS

1. Preheat oven to 450°F.
2. Mix broccoli, cauliflower, and red pepper together in a large bowl. Sprinkle with basil, salt, and black pepper. Toss well.
3. Divide vegetable mixture onto two pieces of aluminum foil. Top each with on ice cube.
4. Bring up sides of foil and fold ends to form a packet, leaving room for heat circulation inside packet.
5. Bake for 20-25 minutes in oven or grill for approximately 15 minutes in covered grill.

Crunchy Brussels Sprouts

This recipe has become a personal family favorite. Roasting the Brussels sprouts browns them nicely, mellowing their strong flavor and providing a nice, crunchy coating.

MAKES 6 SERVINGS

INGREDIENTS

- 1 ½ pounds Brussels sprouts
- 1 tablespoon olive oil
- ¾ teaspoon salt
- ½ teaspoon black pepper

INSTRUCTIONS

1. Preheat oven to 400°F. Prepare a large baking sheet with nonstick spray and set aside.
2. Cut off brown ends of Brussels sprouts and remove any yellow outer leaves.
3. In a medium bowl, mix Brussels sprouts, olive oil, salt, and black pepper.
4. Evenly spread Brussels sprouts on prepared baking sheet.
5. Roast for 35-45 minutes, until crisp on the outside and tender on the inside. Occasionally rotate sprouts to allow even browning.

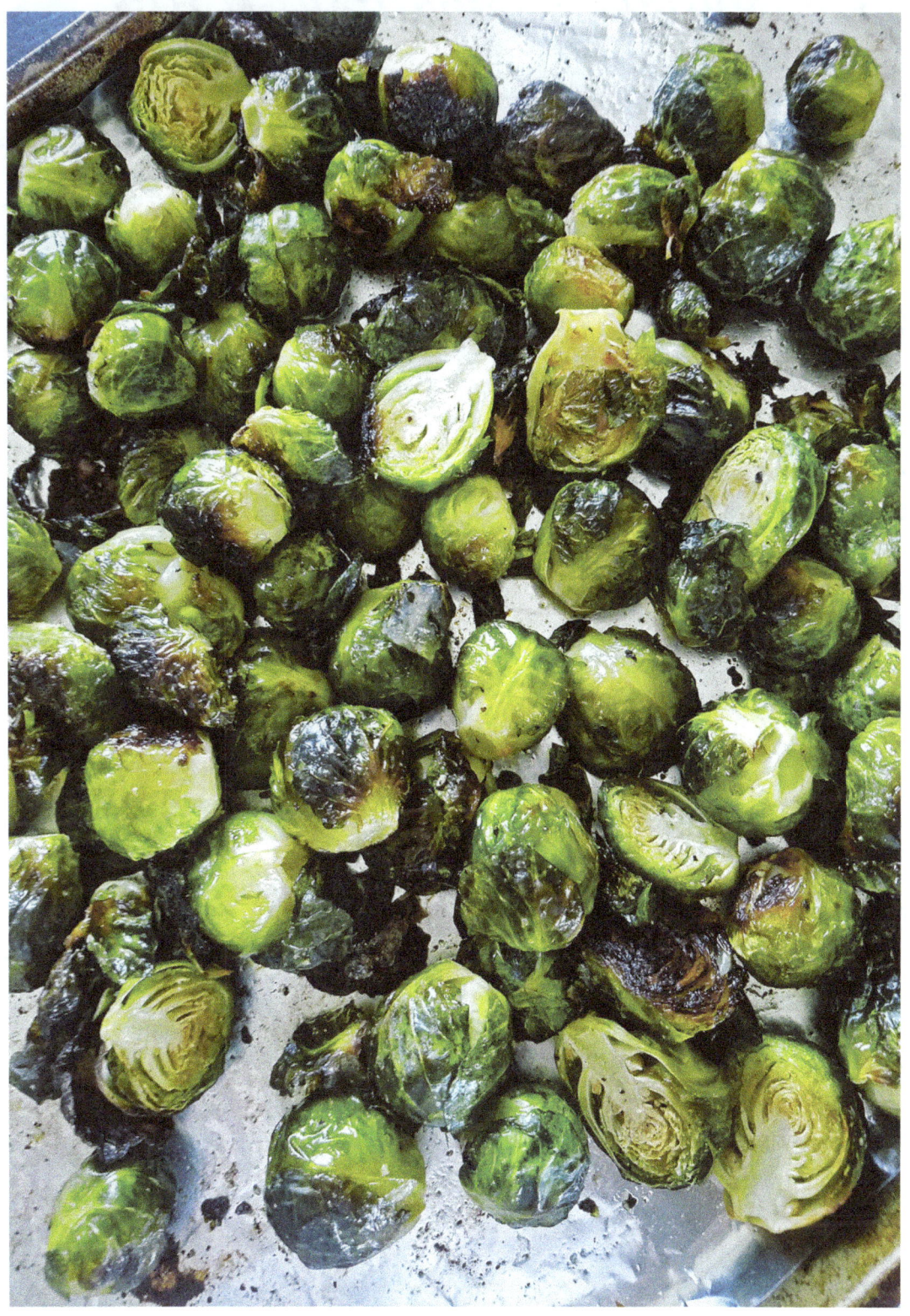

Roasted Vegetable Salad

with Basil Vinaigrette

Potatoes are perfectly highlighted along with several other vegetables in this dish. The honey in the dressing adds just the right amount of sweetness to accompany the rich taste of basil and the other vegetables.

MAKES 6 SERVINGS

INGREDIENTS

- 1 ½ pounds small red potatoes, halved (quartered, if large)
- 12-ounces green beans, cut into 1-inch pieces
- 2 medium red bell peppers, thinly sliced
- 1 red onion, thinly sliced crosswise and separated into rings
- ½ cup low sodium vegetable broth
- 2 cloves garlic
- 2 tablespoons red wine vinegar
- 1 tablespoon honey
- 4 fresh basil leaves, finely chopped
- ½ teaspoon black pepper
- 1 tablespoon lemon juice

INSTRUCTIONS

1. Preheat oven to 425°F. Prepare a 13 x 9-inch baking dish with nonstick spray.
2. Parboil the potatoes for approximately 10-15 minutes.
3. Add the potatoes, green beans, red peppers, red onion, vegetable broth, and garlic to prepared baking dish and mix well.
4. Roast in the oven for 20-30 minutes, stirring every 10 minutes, until the vegetables are tender. Set aside.
5. In a small bowl, whisk together the vinegar, honey, basil, and black pepper.
6. Place the vegetables in a large bowl. Add the dressing and toss to mix well.
7. Sprinkle with the lemon juice before serving.

Hot Sides

Broccoli Soufflé

Soufflés are elegant and delicious but have a reputation of being tricky to make. This fool-proof recipe challenges that notion, allowing you to make a light and fluffy soufflé in your own kitchen. Not only will your guests be impressed by its appearance, it's so delicious that they'll be begging for more!

MAKES 12 SERVINGS

INGREDIENTS

- 2 large heads fresh broccoli, chopped
- 2 tablespoons low fat margarine
- 1 clove garlic, minced
- ½ teaspoon salt
- ¼ teaspoon black pepper
- ¼ cup all-purpose flour
- ½ cup plain soy milk
- 2 tablespoons light mayonnaise
- 1 whole egg
- 3 egg whites, beaten

INSTRUCTIONS

1. Preheat oven to 350°F. Prepare a 9 x 9-inch baking dish with nonstick spray and set aside.
2. Steam broccoli until soft consistency. Set aside.
3. In a saucepan, melt margarine. Stir in garlic, salt, black pepper, and flour until crumbly. Gradually add soy milk and stir until thickened, approximately 2 minutes.
4. Stir in broccoli and mayonnaise and remove from heat. Stir in egg and fold in egg whites.
5. Pour into prepared baking dish and bake for 40 minutes.

Asparagus
with Mustard Vinaigrette

As a simple way to dress up asparagus, this recipe is sure to become a staple side dish for your family meals. The mustard vinaigrette provides a sweet yet salty taste to the asparagus. It is an elegant and easy vegetable to complement a meal while entertaining.

MAKES 8 SERVINGS

INGREDIENTS

- 1 pound fresh asparagus (preferably thin spears)
- 2 teaspoons Dijon mustard
- 3 tablespoons red wine vinegar
- 1 teaspoon sugar
- ¼ teaspoon salt
- ¼ teaspoon black pepper
- 1 tablespoon minced fresh parsley
- 2 tablespoons olive oil

INSTRUCTIONS

1. Wash asparagus and trim ends. If stems are tough, remove the outer layer with a vegetable peeler.
2. Steam asparagus for approximately 8 minutes or until desired texture is reached.
3. In a bowl, whisk together mustard, vinegar, sugar, salt, black pepper, and parsley. Whisk in olive oil until mixture is blended.
4. Pour mixture over cooked asparagus.

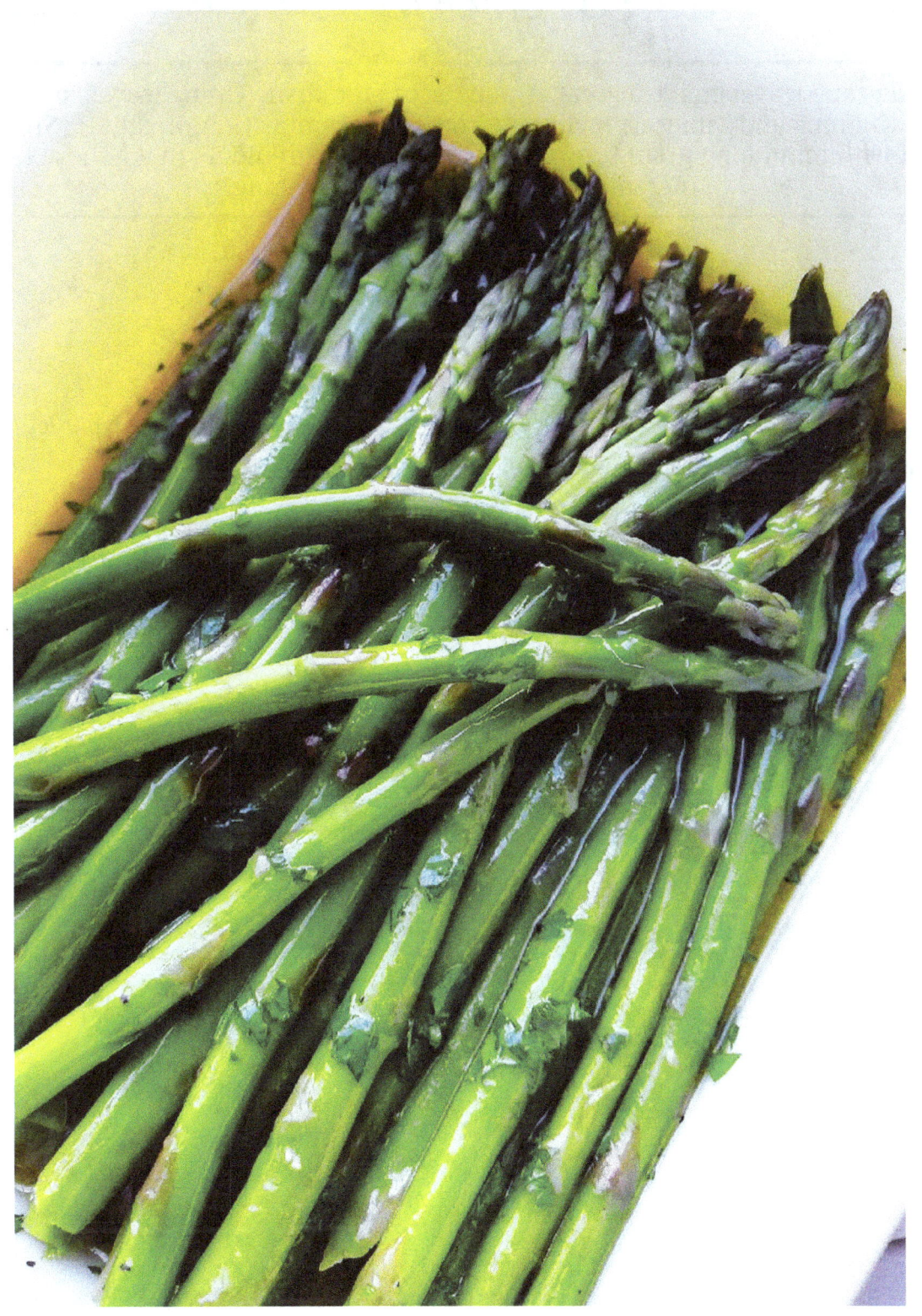

Stuffed Grape Leaves

Stuffed grape leaves make a great appetizer or side dish. Grape leaves are packed with vitamins and minerals including iron and vitamins C, A, K, and E. Stuffing them with mint, long grain brown rice, and other ingredients make these leaves incredibly appetizing and refreshing.

MAKES 7 SERVINGS

INGREDIENTS

- 2 medium onions, chopped
- 3 scallions, chopped
- 1 tablespoon olive oil
- ⅔ cup uncooked long grain brown rice
- 1 ½ cup water
- 1 (8-ounce) can tomato sauce
- 2 tablespoons fresh mint
- 2 tablespoons chopped fresh parsley
- 2 tablespoons fresh basil
- 1 tablespoon ground cinnamon
- 1 teaspoon ground cumin
- 14 grape leaves

INSTRUCTIONS

1. Sauté onions and scallions in olive oil until tender. Add the uncooked rice, water, and tomato sauce and cook until rice is tender.
2. Add the mint, parsley, basil, cinnamon, and cumin.
3. Assemble grape leaves by placing 1 tablespoon of rice mixture into each grape leaf and roll tightly.
4. Place stuffed grape leaves seam side down into large pot. Cover with enough water to cover the bottom of the pan. Cover pan and cook for 20 minutes.

Raisin & Craisin Potato Mounds

Have your children ever asked if they could have dessert for dinner? Well this recipe is a way to please both parent and child when that question is asked. Sweet potatoes are packed with potassium, fiber, and vitamin C. Sweet compromise!

MAKES 12 SERVINGS

INGREDIENTS

- 1 large sweet potato cut into ½-inch pieces
- 1 medium yellow-flesh potato, peeled and cut into ½-inch pieces
- 1 medium onion, chopped
- 2 scallions, finely chopped
- ½ Granny Smith apple, finely chopped
- 1 tablespoon olive oil, divided
- ¼ cup raisins
- ¼ cup craisins
- ⅛ teaspoon salt
- ⅛ teaspoon black pepper
- ⅛ teaspoon ginger
- ⅛ teaspoon dried parsley

INSTRUCTIONS

1. In a large saucepan, boil sweet potatoes and yellow potato pieces until fork-tender, approximately 20 minutes. Drain and set aside.
2. In a nonstick skillet, sauté onion, scallions, and apple in ½ tablespoon of oil for approximately 4-5 minutes. Add to potatoes, then add raisins, and craisins. Season with salt, black pepper, ginger, and parsley.
3. Mix well, slightly mashing potatoes.
4. Heat remaining oil in skillet. Form mounds with 2 tablespoons of mixture and brown for 6 minutes. Turn and continue cooking for an additional 6 minutes.

Portobello Mushroom Sauté

All of the Italian flavors in this recipe are soaked up by the hearty Portobello mushroom. The Parmesan cheese adds the perfect touch of flavor that seals the deal. Mushroom fan or not, this sauté is a must try!

MAKES 8 SERVINGS

INGREDIENTS

- 5 large Portobello mushrooms, sliced with stems removed
- 1 cup sliced white mushrooms
- 1 red onion, chopped
- 1 medium red pepper, chopped
- 2 cups spinach leaves
- 2 tablespoons olive oil
- 1 teaspoon dried thyme
- 1 teaspoon garlic powder
- 2 tablespoons grated Parmesan cheese
- 2 tablespoons chopped fresh parsley

INSTRUCTIONS

1. Thoroughly clean all mushrooms.
2. Sauté mushrooms, onions, peppers, and spinach in olive oil. Season with thyme and garlic powder.
3. Sprinkle with Parmesan cheese and chopped parsley.

Hot Sides

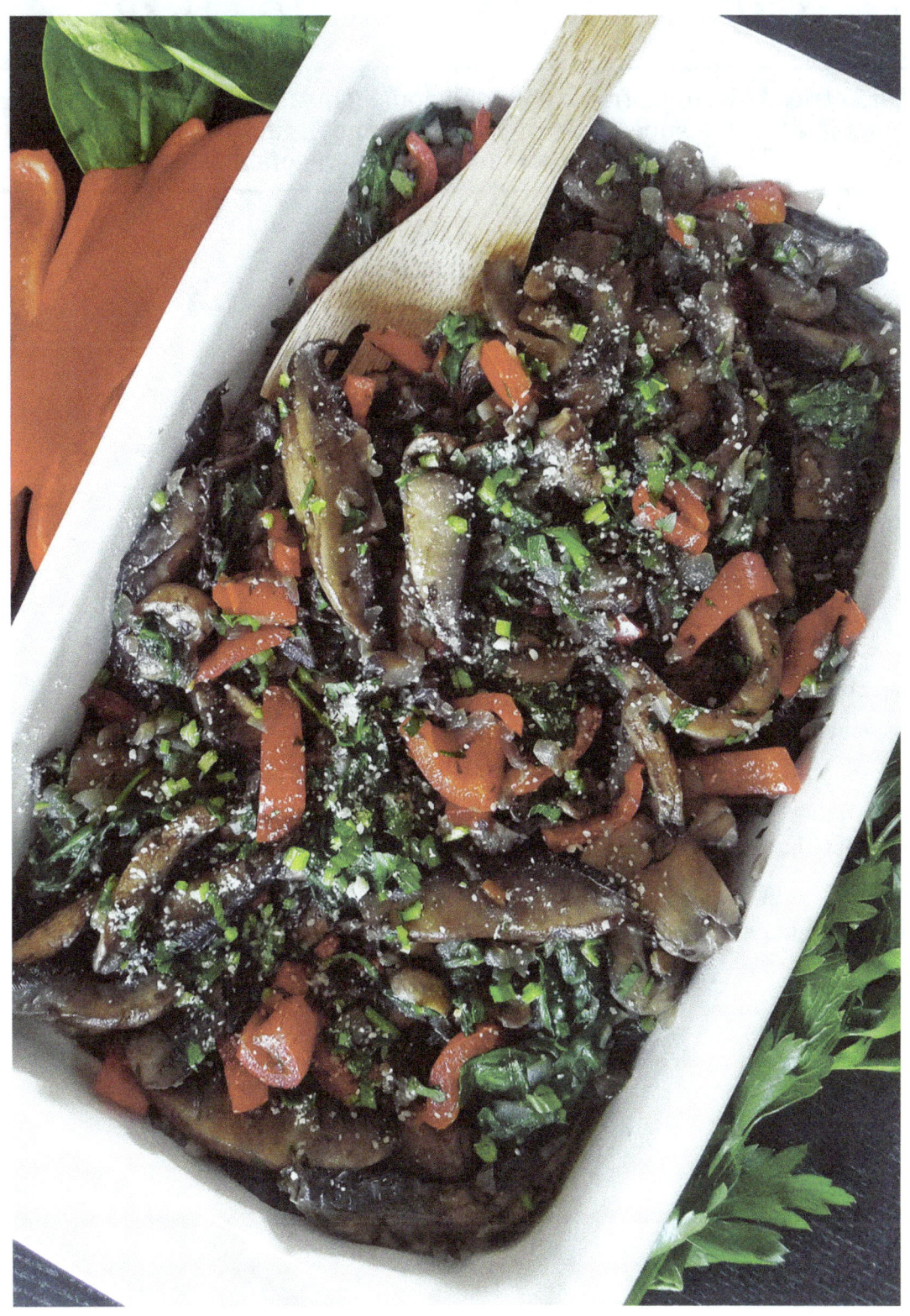

Baked Sweet Potato Fries

Who said fries have to be fried to be delicious? This is a tasty alternative to the traditional fries with a super dose of vitamin A and vitamin C. It's also a great way to get your kids to try a new vegetable!

MAKES 5 SERVINGS

INGREDIENTS

- 4 medium sweet potatoes (approximately 1 pound)
- ½ tablespoon olive oil
- ¼ teaspoon garlic powder
- ¼ teaspoon onion powder
- ⅛ teaspoon paprika

INSTRUCTIONS

1. Preheat oven to 450°F. Prepare a baking sheet with nonstick spray and set aside.
2. Peel sweet potatoes and microwave on HIGH for 5 minutes to soften.
3. Cut sweet potatoes into ½-inch thick sticks, approximately 4-5 inches long.
4. Place potatoes in plastic zip bag. Add olive oil and seasonings and shake well until potatoes are evenly coated.
5. Place potatoes in a single layer on baking sheet.
6. Bake for 20 minutes. Turn potatoes over and return to oven for an additional 20 minutes.

Hot Sides

Stuffed Potato Skins

Craving potato skins but don't enjoy sour cream? For this version, cheddar cheese and white beans provide the same creamy texture. The traditional flavors of green pepper, onion, and garlic powder take this recipe to the next level.

MAKES 12 SERVINGS

INGREDIENTS

- 3 medium Idaho potatoes
- 3 medium sweet potatoes
- 1 medium onion, chopped
- 2 cloves garlic, minced
- 1 medium green bell pepper, chopped
- 1 (5-ounce) can white beans, drained and rinsed
- 1 tablespoon olive oil
- ½ cup shredded low fat Cheddar cheese
- ¼ teaspoon ginger
- ¼ teaspoon garlic powder
- Chopped fresh parsley, for garnish

INSTRUCTIONS

1. Preheat oven to 425°F.
2. Bake potatoes in oven or microwave.
3. Cut potatoes in half. Spoon out potato pulp. Set aside pulp and potato shells for later use.
4. Sauté onions, garlic, green pepper, and white beans in olive oil.
5. Add sautéed mixture to potato pulp. Mix in cheese, ginger, and garlic powder.
6. Fill each potato shell with two tablespoons of the pulp mixture.
7. Garnish each potato skin with parsley.
8. Place on baking sheet and bake for 15 minutes.

Mock Stuffed Derma

This is a very simple dish to make. Once you prepare the rolls, just place it in the oven and set the timer for 50 minutes while you prepare the rest of your meal. You can even bake these in advance and freeze them for a future meal. Children love them too!

MAKES 12 SERVINGS

INGREDIENTS

- 4 medium carrots, grated
- 2 stalks celery, diced
- 1 medium onion, diced
- 8-ounces whole wheat saltine crackers (approximately 4 cups processed)
- 2 tablespoons olive oil, divided
- ½ teaspoon salt
- ¼ teaspoon black pepper

INSTRUCTIONS

1. Preheat oven to 375°F.
2. Combine carrots, celery, onion, saltines, 1 tablespoon olive oil, salt, and black pepper in food processor.
3. Blend, then add remaining oil and process again.
4. Form 2 rolls out of blended mixture.
5. Wrap each roll in foil and bake for 50-60 minutes.

Hot Sides

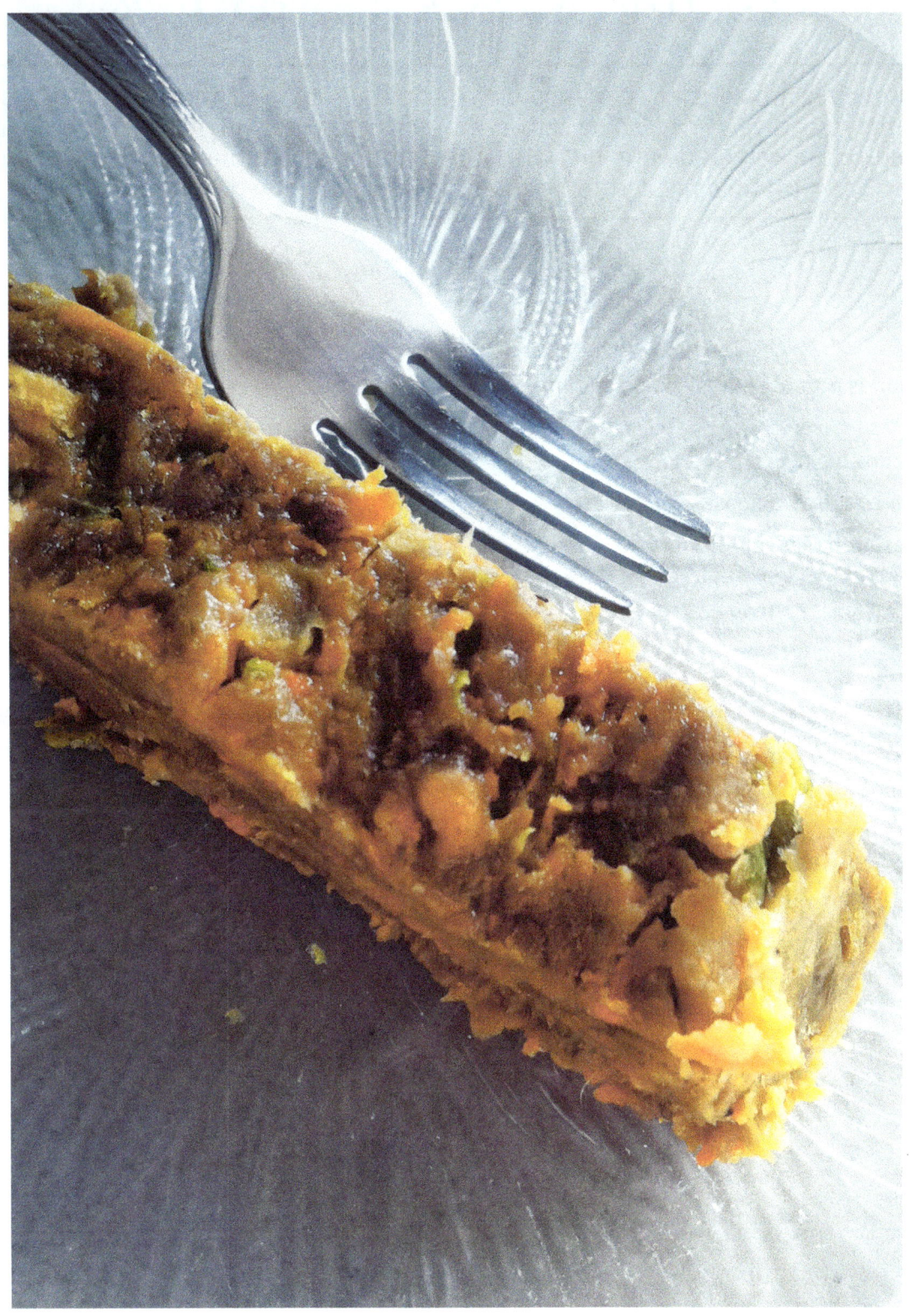

Vibrant Mashed Potatoes

Have you ever mixed the vegetables on your plate into your mashed potatoes after plating your meal? Well this recipe embraces that idea, giving you the creamy mashed potatoes you desire, but with a few added vegetable surprises! Who said potatoes needed to be the only star in mashed potatoes?

MAKES 12 SERVINGS

INGREDIENTS

- 2 pounds potatoes, peeled and cut into chunks
- 1 ½ cups plain soy milk
- 1 cup chopped onions
- 2 teaspoon olive oil
- 1 cup chopped carrots
- 1 cup green beans or snow peas
- 1 cup broccoli florets
- ¼ teaspoon salt
- ¼ teaspoon black pepper

INSTRUCTIONS

1. In a large pot, boil potatoes until soft. Mash potatoes and add soy milk.
2. In a separate pan, sauté onions in olive oil for approximately 5 minutes. Add carrots and cook for another 10 minutes. Add green beans and broccoli until tender.
3. Combine mashed potatoes and vegetables. Heat through and season with salt and black pepper.

Hot Sides

Brown Rice Bake

Brown rice is a great side because it complements a variety of dishes. This recipe adds a little pop to plain brown rice with the addition of spices and tart apples. Say bye-bye to boring rice!

MAKES 8 SERVINGS

INGREDIENTS

- 1 medium red apple, peeled and diced
- 1 small onion, chopped
- 1 stalk celery, chopped
- 1 teaspoon olive oil
- 1 teaspoon garlic powder
- 1 teaspoon onion powder
- ¼ teaspoon thyme
- ¼ teaspoon white pepper
- 3 cups cooked brown rice

INSTRUCTIONS

1. Preheat oven to 350°F. Prepare a baking dish with nonstick spray and set aside.
2. In a nonstick skillet, sauté apple, onion, and celery in olive oil for 5 minutes.
3. Add garlic powder, onion powder, thyme, and pepper. Continue to cook until the vegetables are tender-crisp, approximately 5-10 minutes.
4. Stir in cooked rice, mixing thoroughly.
5. Spread mixture into baking dish and cover tightly. Bake for 25 minutes.

Ginger Caraway Carrots

A warm glaze of olive oil, brown sugar, ginger, and caraway seeds is made to coat tender carrots. This delicious and healthy vegetable side can be made in no time!

MAKES 8 SERVINGS

INGREDIENTS

- 1 tablespoon olive oil
- 1 tablespoon brown sugar
- ¼ teaspoon ground ginger
- ¼ teaspoon caraway seeds
- 1 ½ pounds small carrots (about 16 small carrots), peeled

INSTRUCTIONS

1. Preheat oven to 450°F.
2. Mix olive oil, brown sugar, ginger, and caraway seeds.
3. In a large bowl, toss carrots in the dressing.
4. Transfer to an oven-safe dish, laying carrots in a single layer. Pour any extra dressing over carrots.
5. Bake for 10 minutes. Toss carrots in pan. Return to oven for an additional 10 minutes until carrots tender and beginning to brown.

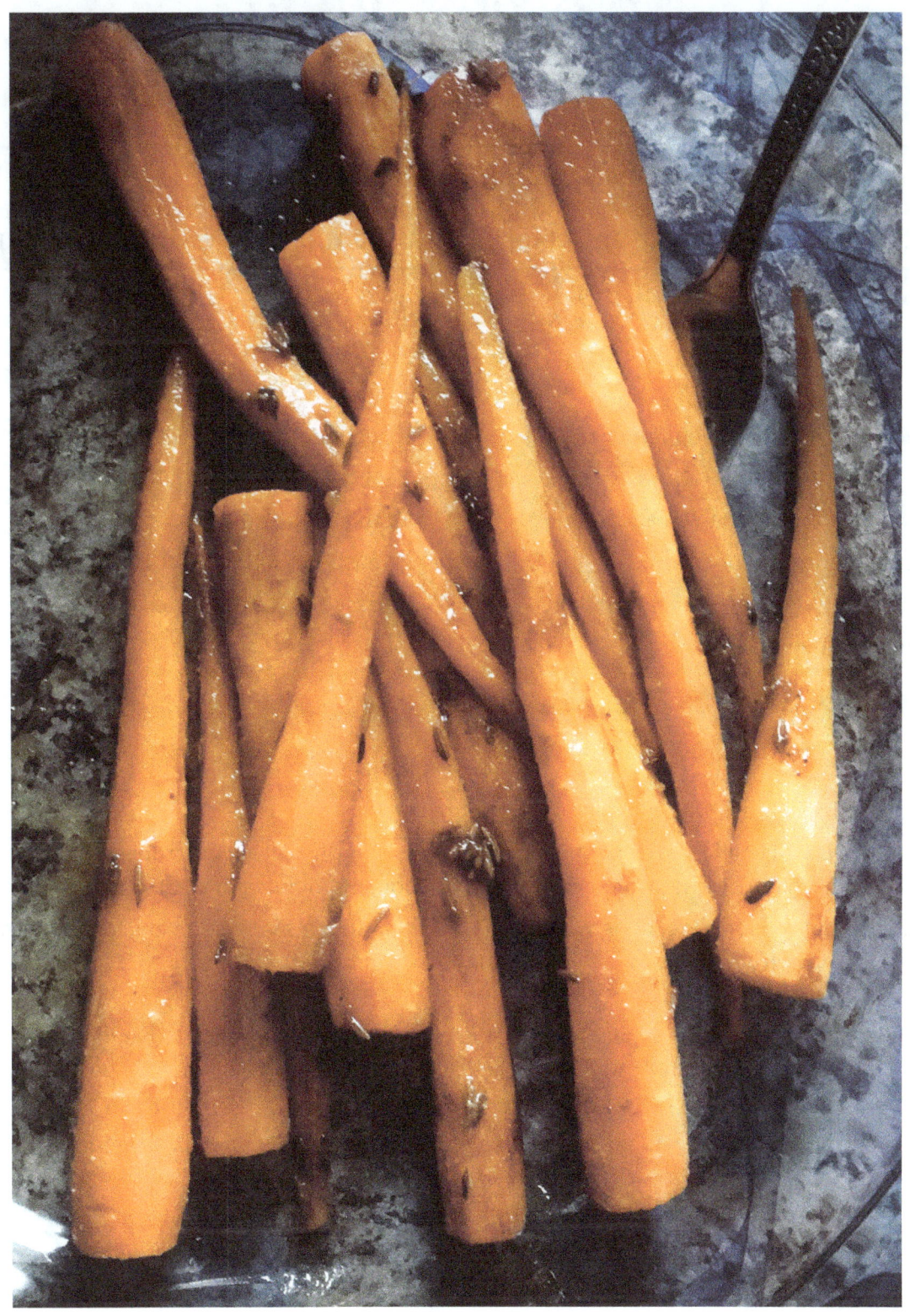

Couscous Salad
with Tomatoes & Roasted Pepper

This recipe shows just how delicious ingredients in their natural form can be. Couscous is a favorite base to Mediterranean dishes. Vegetables and fresh herbs boost the flavor for a fresh and colorful dish you will love serving to your family.

MAKES 8 SERVINGS

INGREDIENTS

- 1 medium yellow bell pepper
- 1 ½ cups water
- 1 cup uncooked whole wheat couscous
- 2 cups diced plum tomatoes
- ½ cup finely chopped flat leaf parsley
- ¼ cup chopped scallions
- ¼ cup low sodium vegetable broth
- 2 tablespoons lemon juice
- 1 tablespoon olive oil
- ½ teaspoon salt
- ¼ teaspoon black pepper

INSTRUCTIONS

1. Prepare a broiler rack with nonstick cooking spray.
2. Cut bell pepper in half lengthwise and remove seeds and ribs. Place on broiler rack, cut sides down. Broil about 3 inches from heat source for about 18 minutes or until skin is blackened.
3. While peppers are broiling, bring water to a boil in a medium saucepan. Add couscous and cover. Remove from heat and let stand 5 minutes or until water is absorbed. Transfer to a large bowl and fluff with a fork
4. Remove bell peppers from broiler and place in a bowl until cool enough to handle. Once cooled, remove and discard the charred skins, then dice peppers. Add roasted pepper, tomatoes, parsley and scallions to the couscous.
5. In a small bowl, whisk vegetable broth, lemon juice, olive oil, salt, and black pepper. Pour over salad and toss to combine.

Spanish Rice

Want to kick up the flavor tonight? This authentic dish will make your taste buds sing. The added bonus is that it's full of fiber, vitamins, and minerals that will make your body feel great. No more boxed rice over here!

MAKES 8 SERVINGS

INGREDIENTS

- 1 cup uncooked brown rice
- 1 medium onion, chopped
- 1 medium green bell pepper, chopped
- 1 teaspoon olive oil
- 2 (8-ounce) cans tomato sauce
- 1 teaspoon onion powder
- 1 teaspoon garlic powder

INSTRUCTIONS

1. Cook rice according to package directions and set aside.
2. While rice is cooking, sauté onion and green pepper in olive oil until soft and translucent.
3. Add sautéed onion and pepper mixture to cooked rice.
4. Add tomato sauce and season with onion and garlic powder.
5. Heat for 10 minutes until heated through.

Penne Pasta
with Spinach & Red Kidney Beans

This pasta dish has a creamy texture from the ricotta cheese and red kidney beans. The spinach adds color, iron, and vitamin A. You could even enjoy this dish as your entrée by adding a side salad for a complete meal.

MAKES 8 SERVINGS

INGREDIENTS

- 1 (8-ounce) box whole wheat penne pasta
- 1 (20-ounce) box frozen chopped spinach, thawed and strained
- 2 cloves garlic
- 1 tablespoon olive oil
- 1 (15-ounce) can red kidney beans, drained and rinsed
- ¼ teaspoon salt
- ½ teaspoon garlic powder
- 1 cup low fat ricotta cheese
- 1 tablespoon lemon juice

INSTRUCTIONS

1. Cook pasta according to package directions and set aside.
2. In a nonstick skillet, sauté spinach and garlic in olive oil.
3. Add the beans and heat approximately 7 minutes. Season with salt and garlic powder. Remove from heat.
4. Add the ricotta cheese. Toss with pasta and lemon juice.

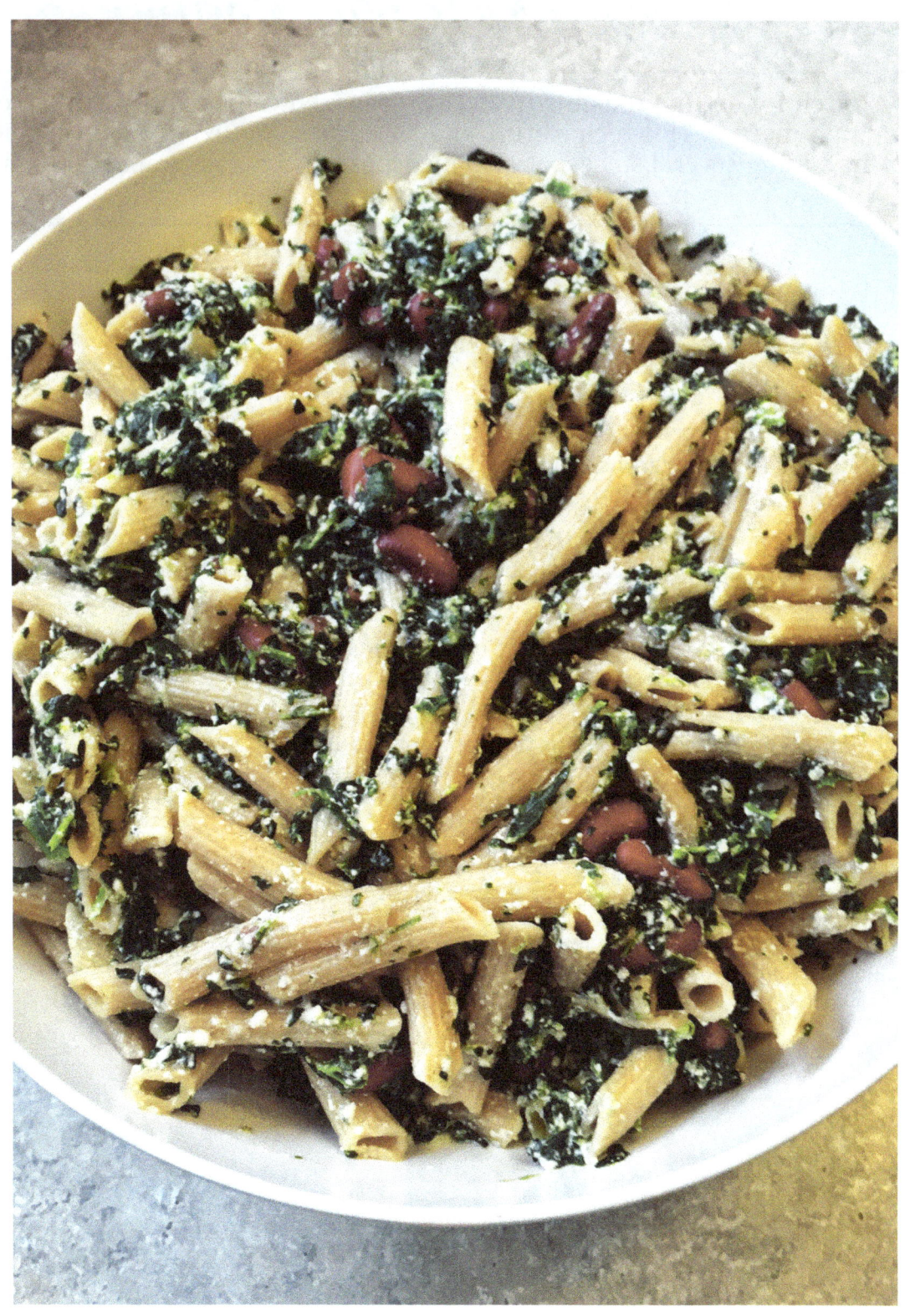

Barley Vegetable Medley

People often forget that the nutritive value of frozen vegetables is the same as fresh, if not better. This recipe brings flavor excitement to a frozen vegetable medley by adding several spices. It also incorporates a whole grain making it the perfect side dish to any lean protein!

MAKES 12 SERVINGS

INGREDIENTS

- 1 cup uncooked barley
- 1 (16-ounce) package frozen vegetable medley (sugar snap peas, carrots, onions and mushrooms)
- ½ cup low sodium vegetable broth
- 1 (8-ounce) can water chestnuts, drained
- 1 teaspoon garlic powder
- 1 tablespoon dried basil
- ½ teaspoon oregano
- ½ teaspoon thyme
- 1 teaspoon lemon pepper

INSTRUCTIONS

1. Cook barley according to package directions and set aside.
2. Cook frozen vegetables in vegetable broth until tender. Remove vegetables and reduce the liquid in the pot to 2 tablespoons.
3. Mix barley with water chestnuts and cooked vegetables and set aside.
4. In a small bowl, combine garlic powder, basil, oregano, thyme, and lemon pepper. Add to broth.
5. Pour mixture over barley and vegetables and mix well. Heat through.

Hot Sides

Curried Brown Rice Salad
with Green Beans

The flavors of the Middle East in this recipe are strong and savory. In each forkful of this side dish, curry and cilantro will dance on your tongue in a symphony of flavors that you're sure to love.

MAKES 12 SERVINGS

INGREDIENTS

- 2 cups water
- 1 cup uncooked long grain brown rice
- 2 cups diagonally cut green beans
- ½ medium red bell pepper, diced
- 1 tablespoon finely chopped cilantro
- 2 tablespoons lemon juice
- 1 tablespoon olive oil
- 1 ½ teaspoons curry powder
- ½ teaspoon salt
- ¼ teaspoon black pepper

INSTRUCTIONS

1. In a large saucepan, combine water and rice. Cover and bring to a boil; reduce heat and simmer 40 minutes or until water is absorbed and rice in tender. Cool to room temperature.
2. Steam beans in a covered steamer basket over boiling water for 5 minutes or until crisp-tender. Rinse under cold water and drain well.
3. In a large bowl, combine rice, beans, red pepper, and cilantro.
4. In a smaller bowl, whisk together lemon juice, olive oil, curry powder, salt, and black pepper. Pour over rice mixture and toss to combine.

Tomato Mushroom Barley Risotto

This risotto recipe is great to make if you want a warm, hearty dish that is full of flavor. The barley absorbs the veggie broth to create a moist, chewy consistency. The mushrooms add texture and protein.

MAKES 8 SERVINGS

INGREDIENTS

- 1 medium onion, chopped
- 2 cloves garlic, minced
- 1 tablespoon olive oil
- 8-ounces sliced fresh mushrooms
- 1 ½ cups uncooked pearl barley
- 4 cups low sodium vegetable broth
- 2 cups diced tomato
- ½ teaspoon salt
- ⅛ teaspoon black pepper
- ½ teaspoon dried thyme or 1 ½ teaspoon chopped fresh thyme
- 2 tablespoons chopped fresh parsley

INSTRUCTIONS

1. Sauté onion and garlic in olive oil until soft.
2. Add mushrooms and cook until brown.
3. Add barley and mix until lightly toasted, approximately 5 minutes.
4. Add vegetable broth, tomato, salt, black pepper, thyme, and parsley.
5. Bring to a boil, cover and simmer for at least 25 minutes. Stir intermittently.

Intuitive Eating Wisdom

Intuitive Eating Principle 2:
Honor Your Hunger

Years of dieting can make it difficult to recognize your hunger signals. Feeling hunger is normal and natural for the body; fueling your body with food provides the energy needed to feel your best. Resisting these natural signals may lead you to feeling ravenous and then overeat. Honor those first signs of hunger, trusting your body to guide you.

Cold Sides

IN THIS CHAPTER

105 | Corn Salad

106 | Edamame Vegetable Salad

108 | Lentil & Red Pepper Salad

109 | Vegetable Orzo

110 | Three Bean Salsa

112 | Mixed Potato Salad

113 | Classic Macaroni Salad

114 | Flavorful Couscous

116 | Bowtie Zucchini Pasta

117 | Wild Rice Pilaf Salad

118 | Tabouli Salad

120 | Wheat Berry Bean Salad

121 | Angel Hair & Cabbage Salad

122 | Greek Rotini Salad

Cold Sides

Corn Salad

Enjoy a sweet side that is colorful and delicious. The sour pickles and the natural sweetness of corn and relish create the perfect blend of flavors. This side dish is great on its own or as an accompaniment to your favorite dishes at a barbecue.

MAKES 12 SERVINGS

INGREDIENTS

- 2 (15-ounce) cans Mexi-corn, drained
- 1 medium tomato, diced
- 2 sour pickles, diced
- 1 small red bell pepper, chopped
- ⅓ cup light mayonnaise
- 2 tablespoons sweet pickle relish
- 1 teaspoon lemon juice
- ½ tablespoon chopped dill

INSTRUCTIONS

1. Mix together corn, tomato, pickles and red pepper. Set aside.
2. In a separate bowl, mix mayonnaise, relish, and lemon juice.
3. Pour dressing into corn mixture and toss to coat. Add chopped dill and mix.
4. Chill in refrigerator for 1 hour.

Edamame Vegetable Salad

This is a great dish to make in advance so that the vegetables absorb the flavors. Edamame has gained popularity as they are an excellent source of vegetable protein, dietary fiber, and iron and a unique base to use for a salad. The wide variety of vegetables that are incorporated provide even more nutrients to this Asian-inspired dish.

MAKES 6 SERVINGS

INGREDIENTS

- 2 cups fresh or frozen edamame kernels
- ½ cup chopped artichoke hearts
- 3 cups thinly sliced red cabbage
- 1 cup shredded carrots
- 2 scallions, chopped
- 2 stalks celery, diced
- 3 tablespoons rice vinegar
- 1 tablespoon sesame oil
- 1 teaspoon low sodium soy sauce

INSTRUCTIONS

1. Combine the edamame, artichoke hearts, red cabbage, carrots, scallions, and celery.
2. In a separate bowl, whisk together rice vinegar, sesame oil, and soy sauce.
3. Pour dressing over edamame vegetable mixture and toss well.
4. Refrigerate several hours or overnight.

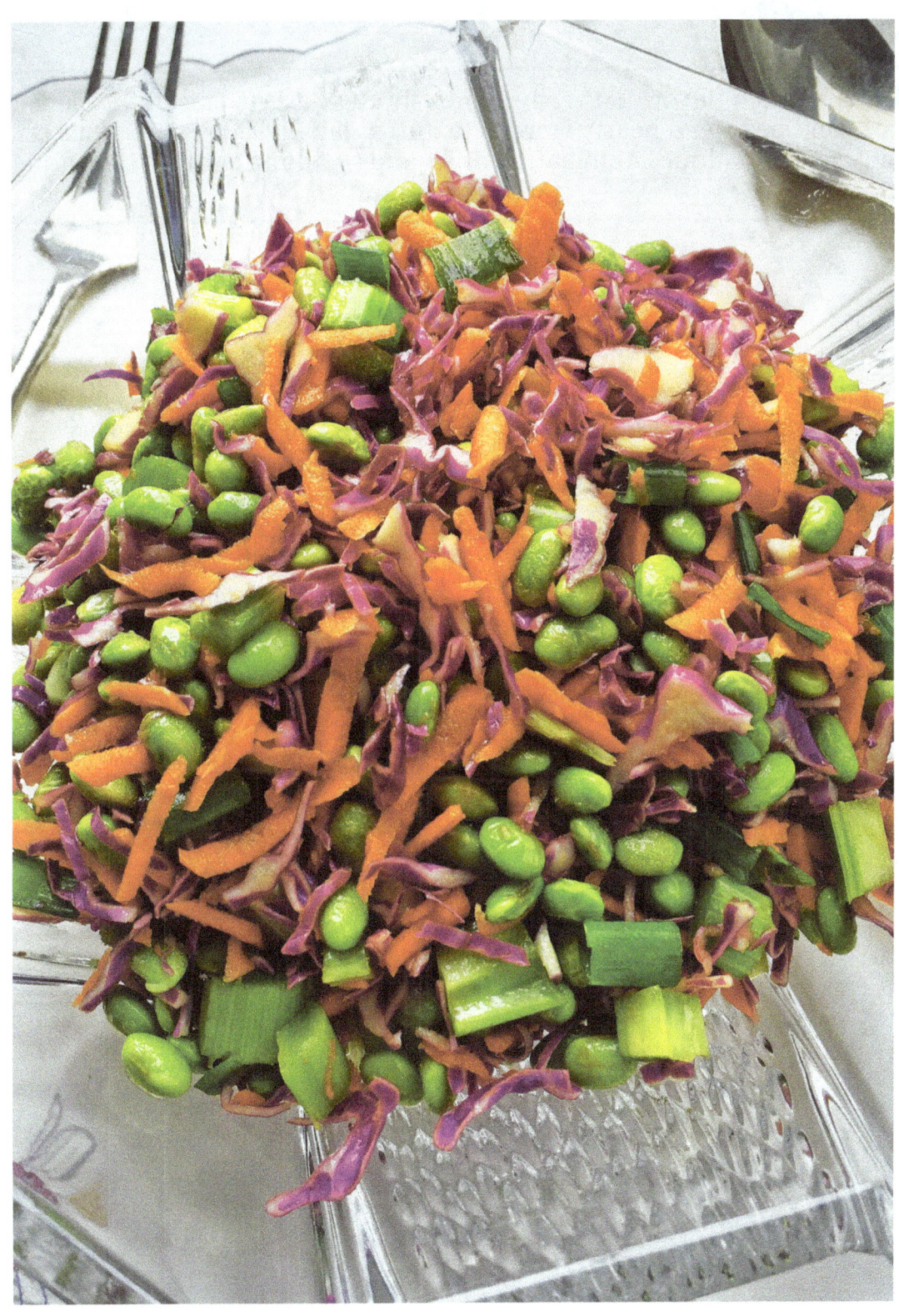

Lentil & Red Pepper Salad

Lentils have a rich flavor that really comes through as the star in this salad. The potatoes and peas lend hearty starchy textures to balance out the other crunchy vegetables. This unique combination of legumes will make this a crowd-pleasing favorite for sure!

MAKES 8 SERVINGS

INGREDIENTS

- 2 cups cooked lentils
- 1 cup diced cooked potatoes
- ½ cup frozen green peas
- ½ cup finely chopped red bell pepper
- ¼ cup chopped red onion
- ¼ cup chopped celery
- 1 tablespoon finely chopped fresh parsley
- 1 tablespoon finely chopped basil
- 2 tablespoons red wine vinegar
- 2 tablespoons olive oil
- ⅛ teaspoon salt
- ⅛ teaspoon black pepper

INSTRUCTIONS

1. Combine the lentils, potatoes, peas, red peppers, red onion, celery, parsley, and basil in a large bowl.
2. In a separate bowl, whisk the vinegar, olive oil, salt, and black pepper.
3. Add to the lentil mixture. Toss and serve.
4. Chill in the refrigerator for 2 hours.

Cold Sides

Vegetable Orzo

Orzo is a pasta that is similar to rice but a little heartier. It has a real affinity for absorbing the flavors it's cooked with and this dish is no exception. Loaded with vegetables, this recipe is sure to put a smile on any pasta lover's face!

MAKES 12 SERVINGS

INGREDIENTS

- 1 large onion, diced
- 1 small eggplant, peeled and cubed
- 1 small red bell pepper, chopped
- 1 small yellow bell pepper, chopped
- 1 cup uncooked orzo
- 4 cups low sodium chicken or vegetable broth
- 1 cup water
- 1 (10-ounce) box frozen chopped spinach, thawed and strained
- 1-ounce chopped sun dried tomatoes
- 1 teaspoon garlic powder
- ½ cup chopped fresh basil
- ¼ teaspoon black pepper

INSTRUCTIONS

1. In a large saucepan, sauté onion, eggplant, and peppers until tender.
2. Mix in orzo and cook until slightly browned, approximately 7-10 minutes.
3. Stir in broth and water and bring to a boil until all liquid is absorbed by the orzo.
4. Add chopped spinach and sun dried tomatoes.
5. Season with garlic powder, basil, and black pepper.

Three Bean Salsa

This versatile salsa salad is great because it's vegetable-rich. Enjoy with whole grain chips as a side dish or meal starter, or add grilled chicken or baked fish to make it a main course. The possibilities are yours to discover!

MAKES 12 SERVINGS

INGREDIENTS

- 1 (15-ounce) can dark red kidney beans, drained and rinsed
- 1 (15-ounce) can black beans, drained and rinsed
- 1 (15-ounce) can garbanzo beans, drained and rinsed
- 1 ½ cups steamed sliced carrots
- 1 red onion, diced
- 1 large tomato, chopped
- 1 cup frozen corn niblets
- ¾ cup salsa
- 2 tablespoons olive oil
- 2 tablespoons lime juice
- ½ teaspoon chili powder
- ¼ teaspoon ground cumin

INSTRUCTIONS

1. In a large bowl, combine beans, carrots, red onion, tomato, and corn and set aside.
2. In a separate bowl, combine salsa, olive oil, lime juice, chili powder, and cumin.
3. Pour dressing mixture over bean salad and chill for at least 4 hours.

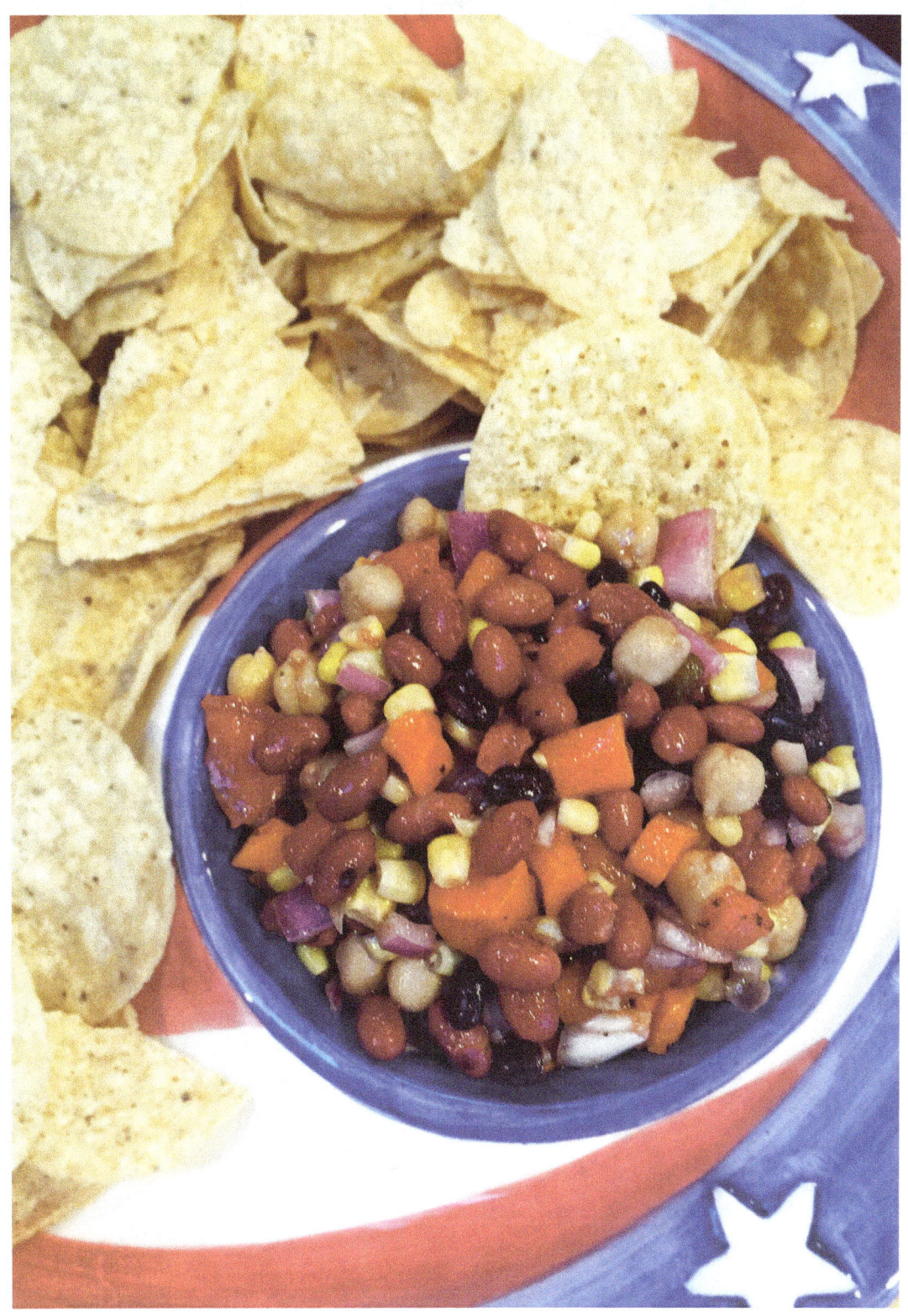

Mixed Potato Salad

This potato salad has a slight twist with sweet potato added for a delicious surprise. Yogurt and Italian dressing make this delightfully creamy and flavorful. The spicy spark added by the nutmeg and curry makes this unlike any potato salad you've picked up from the deli counter.

MAKES 12 SERVINGS

INGREDIENTS

- 1 pound red potatoes
- 1 large sweet potato
- 2 stalks celery, diced
- ½ green bell pepper, chopped
- ½ red bell pepper, chopped
- 2 scallions, chopped
- 1 small red onion, diced
- ½ cup light Italian dressing
- 1 cup plain nonfat yogurt
- 2 tablespoons lemon juice
- 1 teaspoon Dijon mustard
- 1 tablespoon chopped fresh dill
- ½ teaspoon ground nutmeg
- ½ teaspoon curry powder
- ¼ teaspoon black pepper

INSTRUCTIONS

1. Cook the red and sweet potatoes until tender. Drain and let cool. Cut into cubes.
2. In a large bowl, combine the potatoes, chopped celery, bell peppers, scallions, and red onion.
3. In a separate bowl, combine the Italian dressing, yogurt, lemon juice, Dijon mustard, dill, nutmeg, curry powder, and black pepper. Pour over potatoes and toss well to coat.
4. Chill at least 2 hours before serving.

Classic Macaroni Salad

Picnics, barbeques, and tailgates are never complete without a macaroni salad. The Dijon mustard provides the classic creaminess plus extra flavor that is irresistible. This is sure to become your go-to macaroni salad!

MAKES 10 SERVINGS

INGREDIENTS

- 1 (8-ounce) box whole wheat elbow macaroni
- 1 cup sliced celery
- 1 cup chopped red bell pepper
- 1 cup chopped green bell pepper
- ¼ cup chopped onion
- ½ cup light mayonnaise
- 2 tablespoons vinegar
- 1 tablespoon Dijon mustard
- 1 teaspoon sugar
- 1 teaspoon salt
- ¼ teaspoon black pepper

INSTRUCTIONS

1. Cook elbow macaroni according to package directions and place in a large mixing bowl.
2. Add celery, peppers, and onion to macaroni.
3. In a separate bowl, mix mayonnaise, vinegar, Dijon mustard, sugar, salt, and black pepper until a smooth consistency.
4. Add mayonnaise mixture to the macaroni and toss well to coat.
5. Cover and chill before serving.

Flavorful Couscous

The colors and textures really bring this dish to life. Tons of veggies lend all their natural flavors and the golden raisins and ginger add unexpected pops of sweetness to this tantalizing side.

MAKES 14 SERVINGS

INGREDIENTS

- 3 cups low sodium vegetable broth
- ½ teaspoon ground ginger
- 1 ½ cups uncooked couscous
- ¼ cup minced fresh parsley
- ½ teaspoon salt
- 1 cup finely diced carrots
- 1 medium red onion, chopped
- 1 cup finely diced celery
- 1 medium red bell pepper, chopped
- 1 cup chopped broccoli
- 1 tablespoon lemon juice
- ⅓ cup golden raisins

INSTRUCTIONS

1. Put vegetable broth and ginger in a pot and bring to a boil.
2. Add couscous to the pot and reduce heat.
3. Simmer for 20 minutes. Cook until liquid is absorbed, then remove from heat.
4. Add parsley and salt. Fluff couscous with a fork, removing clumps.
5. Let couscous cool for approximately 5 minutes. Once cooled, add carrots, red onion, celery, red pepper, and broccoli and mix well.
6. Add lemon juice and raisins and toss.
7. Chill in refrigerator prior to serving.

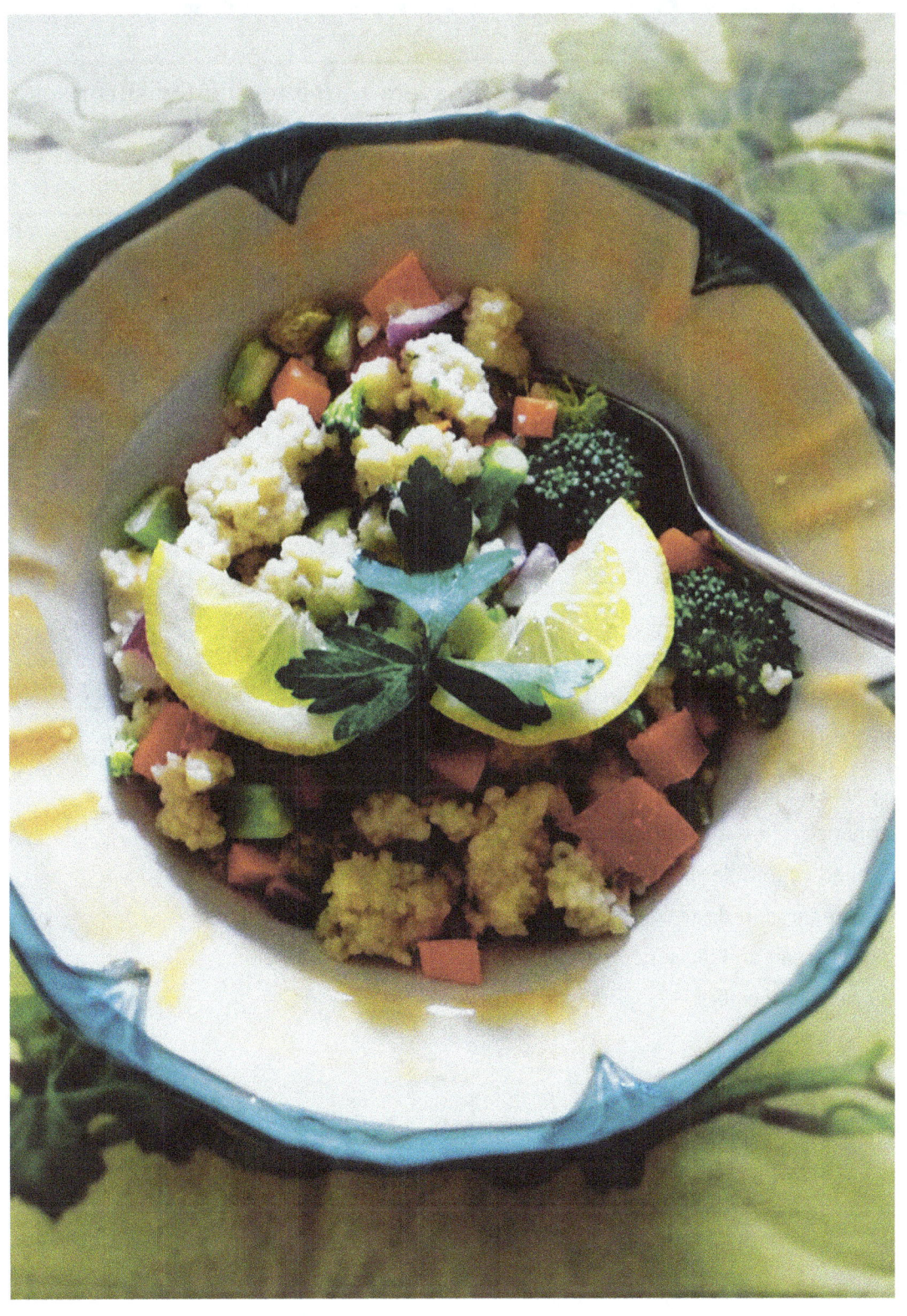

Bowtie Zucchini Pasta

Think of this salad as a cold pasta primavera with a few added surprises. The savory and sweet taste of the sun-dried tomatoes and fresh cherry tomatoes combined with garlic and basil lend classic Italian flavors that are kicked up another notch with the addition of eggplant and zucchini.

MAKES 25 SERVINGS

INGREDIENTS

- 1 (16-ounce) box whole wheat bowtie pasta
- 1 medium zucchini, peeled and sliced
- 1 small eggplant, peeled and diced
- 1 medium onion, chopped
- 1 clove garlic
- 1 tablespoon olive oil
- 2 tablespoons balsamic vinegar
- ½ cup chopped sun dried tomatoes
- 20 cherry tomatoes, halved
- 1 tablespoon lemon juice
- ¼ teaspoon salt
- ¼ teaspoon black pepper
- ¼ cup chopped fresh basil

INSTRUCTIONS

1. Cook pasta according to package directions and set aside.
2. In a nonstick pan, sauté zucchini, eggplant, onion and garlic in olive oil.
3. Stir cooked vegetables into pasta.
4. Mix in vinegar, sun-dried tomatoes, cherry tomatoes, and lemon juice.
5. Season with salt and black pepper. Add chopped basil and mix well.
6. Refrigerate until chilled.

Cold Sides

Wild Rice Pilaf Salad

The rice isn't the only thing wild about this recipe! Dill weed and dry mustard give it a flavor boost that complements the freshness of the vegetables for a wildly delicious side to any meal!

MAKES 20 SERVINGS

INGREDIENTS

- 2 cups uncooked wild rice pilaf
- 1 large carrot, chopped
- 1 (14 ½-ounce) can corn niblets
- 2 scallions, sliced
- 2 cucumbers, chopped
- ⅓ cup chopped fresh parsley
- ⅓ cup olive oil
- ¼ cup lemon juice
- ½ teaspoon dill weed
- ¼ teaspoon dry mustard
- ¼ teaspoon black pepper
- 2 cloves garlic, chopped

INSTRUCTIONS

1. Cook wild rice pilaf according to package directions.
2. Mix carrots, corn, scallions, cucumbers, and parsley in a bowl, then mix into rice.
3. In a separate bowl, combine olive oil, lemon juice, dill weed, dry mustard, black pepper, and garlic.
4. Mix into rice and vegetables and toss well.
5. Serve warm or cold.

Tabouli Salad

This salad has such a unique taste. It contains bulgur, a whole grain that is a great source of dietary fiber and protein. With spinach and peppers added, it has even more nutrients. The mint and parsley blend perfectly with the vegetables. Try it as is or with whole grain crackers.

MAKES 9 SERVINGS

INGREDIENTS

- 1 cup uncooked bulgur
- 1 ½ cups boiling water
- 3 cloves garlic, finely chopped
- ½ cup chopped baby spinach
- ½ red bell pepper, chopped
- ½ yellow bell pepper, chopped
- ½ tomato, chopped
- 1 small onion, chopped
- 1 cup chopped fresh parsley
- ½ cup chopped mint
- ½ cucumber, chopped
- ½ cup lemon juice
- 4 tablespoons olive oil
- ¼ teaspoon black pepper
- ¼ teaspoon ground cinnamon

INSTRUCTIONS

1. Place bulgur in a large heatproof bowl. Add the boiling water and cover. Let sit about 30 minutes, or until water is absorbed.
2. Fluff the cooked bulgur with a fork to loosen. Add the garlic, spinach, bell pepper, tomato, onion, parsley, mint, and cucumber and combine.
3. In a separate bowl, whisk together lemon juice, olive oil, black pepper, and cinnamon. Add to tabouli and toss well.
4. Refrigerate for at least 1 hour.

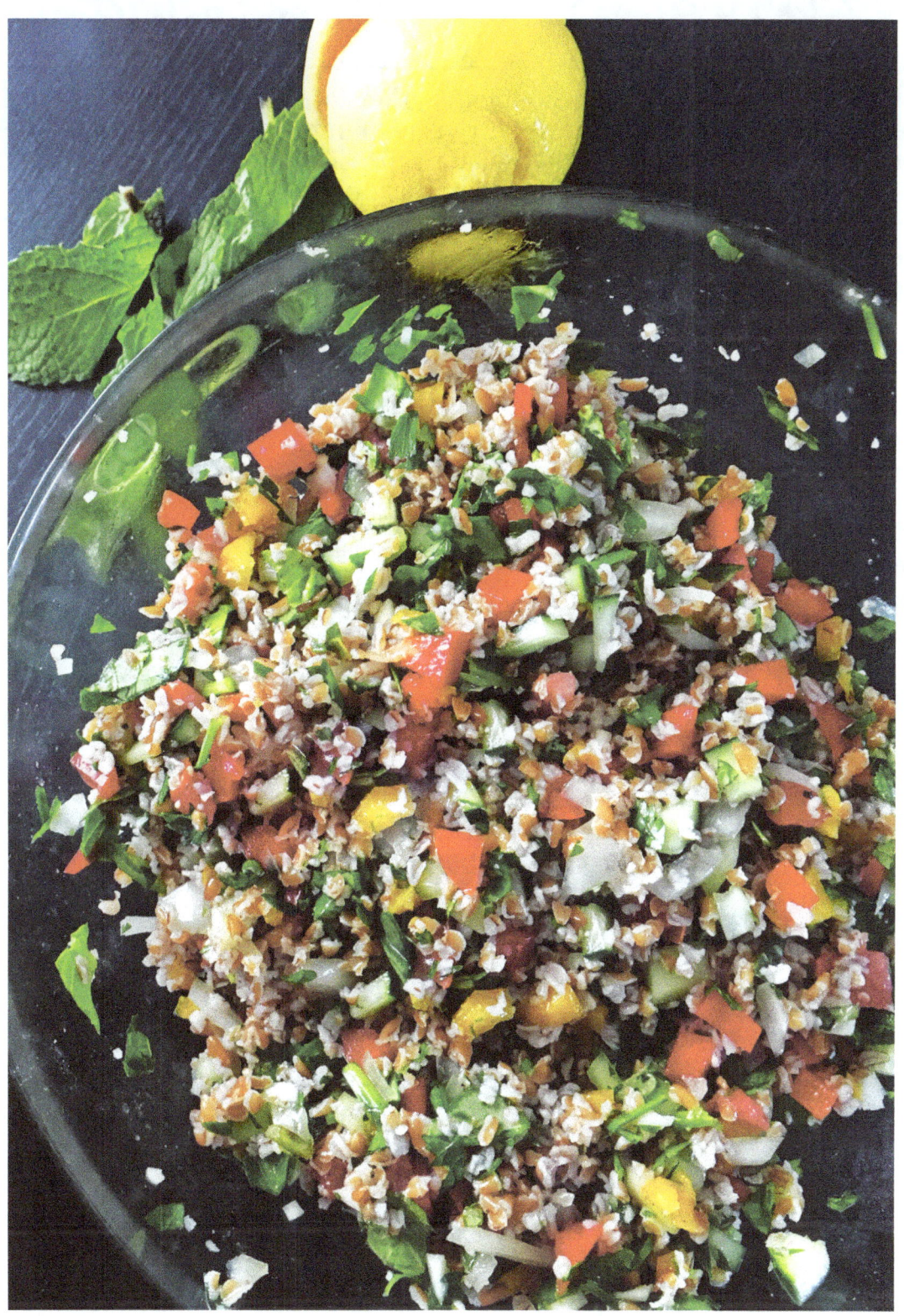

Wheat Berry Bean Salad

This whole grain dish packs a whopping 5 grams of dietary fiber in only a ½ cup serving. The not-so-common wheat berry is high in protein and iron, and makes a lovely and unique base to this bean salad recipe. This revamped classic will leave you wanting to cook with wheat berry more often!

MAKES 24 SERVINGS

INGREDIENTS

- 2 cups uncooked wheat berries
- 1 shallot, chopped
- 1 clove garlic, chopped
- 1 teaspoon olive oil
- ½ teaspoon ground cumin
- 1 (15-ounce) can red kidney beans, drained and rinsed
- 1 (15-ounce) can garbanzo beans, drained and rinsed
- 1 (15-ounce) can pinto beans, drained and rinsed
- 1 small cucumber, diced
- 1 large tomato, diced
- 1 tablespoon lemon juice
- 1 teaspoon chopped mint

INSTRUCTIONS

1. Cook wheat berries according to package directions; cool to room temperature.
2. Sauté shallot and garlic in olive oil. Add cumin and sauté for 8 minutes until shallot is soft and golden brown.
3. Transfer sautéed shallots and garlic to a bowl and mix in beans, cucumber, and tomato.
4. Combine wheat berries with bean and vegetable mixture.
5. Add lemon juice and mint and mix thoroughly.
6. Serve warm or chilled.

Cold Sides

Angel Hair & Red Cabbage Salad

Give a makeover to the traditional elbow macaroni pasta salads and try out this delicious twist that uses angel hair pasta. The red cabbage and vinegar are reminiscent of coleslaw so it's like you get two of your favorite classics in one!

MAKES 12 SERVINGS

INGREDIENTS

- 1 (13-ounce) box whole wheat angel hair pasta
- 2 cups shredded red cabbage
- 1 bunch scallions, sliced
- ⅓ cup olive oil
- ½ cup balsamic vinegar
- ⅓ cup sugar
- 4 tablespoons raisins
- Salt, to taste
- Black pepper, to taste

INSTRUCTIONS

1. Cook pasta according to package directions.
2. Add cabbage and scallions to pasta and mix well.
3. In a separate bowl, whisk together olive oil, balsamic vinegar, and sugar. Toss with pasta.
4. Add raisins and season with salt and black pepper. Mix well.
5. Chill in refrigerator for 2 hours before serving.

Greek Rotini Salad

Do you love the flavors of a Greek salad but feel like it's not filling enough for dinner? The addition of whole wheat pasta plus the creaminess from two cheeses and yogurt is a tasty, filling alternative to traditional Greek Salad.

MAKES 12 SERVINGS

INGREDIENTS

- 1 (16-ounce) box whole wheat rotini
- 1 large tomato, diced
- 1 cucumber, chopped
- ½ cup feta cheese
- ½ cup plain nonfat yogurt
- ½ cup low fat cottage cheese
- ½ cup sliced scallions
- 1 tablespoon chopped dill
- 1 teaspoon garlic powder
- ⅛ teaspoon black pepper
- 2 tablespoons sliced almonds

INSTRUCTIONS

1. Cook pasta according to package directions. Let cool for at least 5 minutes.
2. Add tomato, cucumber, and feta cheese to pasta and set aside.
3. In a blender, combine yogurt, cottage cheese, scallions, dill, garlic powder, and black pepper and blend until smooth. Chill in refrigerator for at least 30 minutes. Pour over pasta and mix well.
4. Sprinkle with sliced almonds

Intuitive Eating Wisdom

Intuitive Eating Principle 3:
Make Peace with Food

Go ahead and eat that piece of chocolate cake! Restricting foods you love causes feelings of deprivation and intense cravings which leads to overindulging, followed by feelings of guilt. Let go of restrictions and give yourself the freedom to eat when you are hungry and enjoy the foods you love.

Kugels & Latkes

IN THIS CHAPTER

127 | Sweet Noodle Kugel

128 | Salt & Pepper Noodle Kugel

130 | Carrot & Parsnip Latkes

131 | Vegetable Kugel

132 | Potato Latkes

134 | Sweet Potato & Apple Latkes

135 | Crisp Potato Kugel

136 | Carrot Kugel

138 | Spinach Noodle Kugel

139 | Pineapple Kugel

Sweet Noodle Kugel

The flavors of raisin, cinnamon and unsweetened applesauce combine perfectly with the hearty texture of whole wheat noodles to provide a nutritious sweet side dish your kids will love!

MAKES 16 SERVINGS

INGREDIENTS

- 1 (12-ounce) package uncooked medium whole wheat noodles
- ¼ cup sugar
- Ground cinnamon
- 1 whole egg
- 2 egg whites
- 2 cups unsweetened applesauce
- ¼ cup raisins

INSTRUCTIONS

1. Preheat oven to 350°F. Prepare a 9 x 13-inch pan with nonstick spray and set aside.
2. Cook noodles according to package directions. Transfer to a large bowl.
3. Mix the sugar with enough cinnamon so the mixture is a rich brown.
4. Beat the egg and egg whites until frothy.
5. Add the cinnamon-sugar mixture, beaten eggs, applesauce, and raisins to the noodles. Mix well.
6. Pour noodles into prepared pan and bake for 45 minutes or until noodles on top are crisp and brown.

Salt & Pepper Noodle Kugel

This kugel is a simple yet tasty dish that pairs well alongside lean meat and roasted veggies to provide a satisfying and well balanced meal.

MAKES 16 SERVINGS

INGREDIENTS

- 1 (12-ounce) package uncooked thin egg noodles
- 1 whole egg, beaten
- 4 egg whites, beaten
- 2 tablespoons olive oil
- 1 teaspoon salt
- 1 ¼ teaspoons black pepper

INSTRUCTIONS

1. Preheat oven to 350°F. Prepare a 9 x 13-inch baking dish with nonstick spray and set aside.
2. Cook noodles according to package directions.
3. Add beaten egg, egg whites, and oil. Mix well. Add salt and black pepper.
4. Pour noodles into prepared pan and bake for approximately 45 minutes or until noodles are crisp and brown.

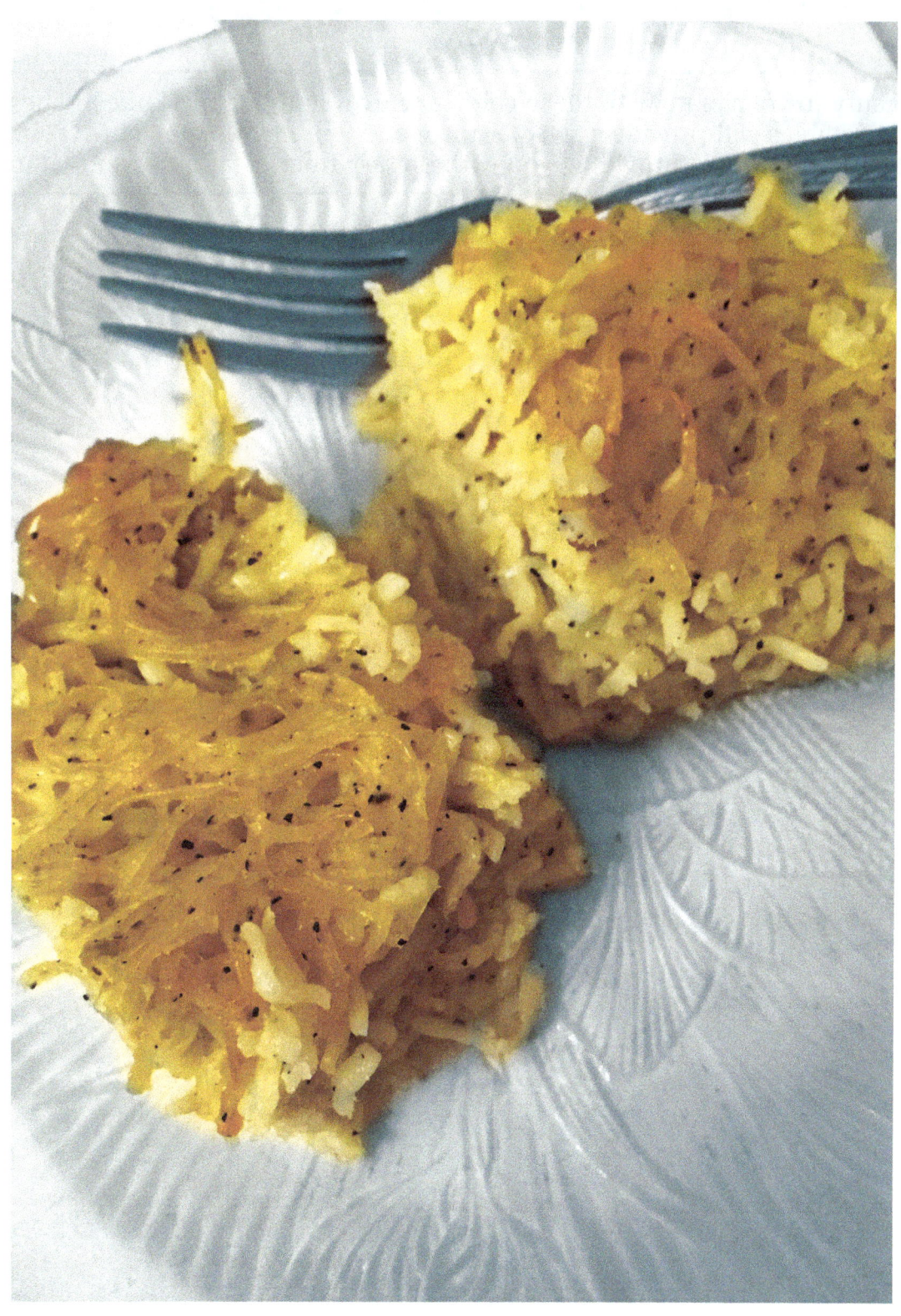

Carrot & Parsnip Latkes

Add beauty to your plate with these colorful carrot and parsnip latkes! These two root vegetables will provide a sweeter taste and lighter color to your traditional potato latke while also providing you with dietary fiber, vitamin A, and vitamin C.

MAKES 12 SERVINGS

INGREDIENTS

- 3 medium to large carrots, peeled and coarsely shredded
- 3 medium parsnips, peeled and coarsely shredded
- 2 teaspoons lemon juice
- 1 egg
- 3 egg whites
- 2 scallions, finely chopped
- ¼ cup all-purpose flour
- ½ teaspoon curry powder
- ½ teaspoon salt
- ¼ teaspoon black pepper
- 1 teaspoon olive oil

INSTRUCTIONS

1. In a large bowl, combine carrots, parsnips, and lemon juice.
2. Beat egg and egg whites. Add to carrot mixture.
3. Add scallions, flour, curry powder, salt, and black pepper and mix thoroughly.
4. Heat oil in nonstick skillet. Drop mixture by 2 tablespoons into pan.
5. Cook over medium-heat until golden brown on both sides.

Vegetable Kugel

This kugel incorporates a variety of delicious vegetables like onions, spinach, carrots, and zucchini to add flavor, texture, and nutrients. This is a fun alternative to simple sautéed vegetables that will definitely become one of your go-to recipes!

MAKES 20 SERVINGS

INGREDIENTS

- 2 medium onions, chopped
- 2 teaspoons olive oil
- 1 (16-ounce) box frozen spinach, thawed and strained
- 2 medium carrots, grated
- 1 medium zucchini, grated
- 1 whole egg
- 2 egg whites
- 2 tablespoons light mayonnaise
- ¼ cup bread crumbs
- ½ teaspoon salt
- ½ teaspoon black pepper
- 1 teaspoon garlic powder
- 1 teaspoon onion powder

INSTRUCTIONS

1. Preheat oven to 350°F. Prepare a 9 x 13-inch baking dish with nonstick spray and set aside.
2. Sauté onion in olive oil.
3. Mix spinach, carrots, and zucchini with sautéed onions.
4. Add egg, egg whites, mayonnaise, and bread crumbs. Mix well.
5. Season with salt, black pepper, garlic powder, and onion powder.
6. Pour into prepared dish and bake for approximately 45 minutes.

Potato Latkes

This recipe is a traditional holiday dish with just a few ingredients that pack all the flavor and crunch you desire from a classic potato latke. Top them off with sour cream, applesauce, or any other family favorite!

MAKES 8 SERVINGS

INGREDIENTS

- 4 medium potatoes (approximately 2 pounds), peeled and coarsely shredded
- 1 medium onion, coarsely grated
- 4 scallions, chopped
- 2 egg whites, beaten
- 2 tablespoons all-purpose flour
- ½ teaspoon salt
- ⅛ teaspoon black pepper
- 1 teaspoon olive oil

INSTRUCTIONS

1. In a large bowl, mix potatoes and onion.
2. Wrap mixture in paper towels and squeeze out all liquid over large measuring cup, placing the mixture in a separate bowl as you go. Potato starch will settle to bottom of measuring cup. Slowly pour off and discard liquid, reserving potato starch.
3. Add scallions, egg whites, flour, salt, black pepper, and reserved potato starch to the potato mixture.
4. Coat nonstick 12-inch skillet with olive oil and heat over medium-high heat.
5. With hands, press together about 2 tablespoons potato mixture; place in skillet and flatten with wide metal spatula. Repeat with remaining potato mixture.
6. Cook pancakes about 8 minutes, turning once, until browned on both sides. Reduce heat if pancakes are browning too quickly.

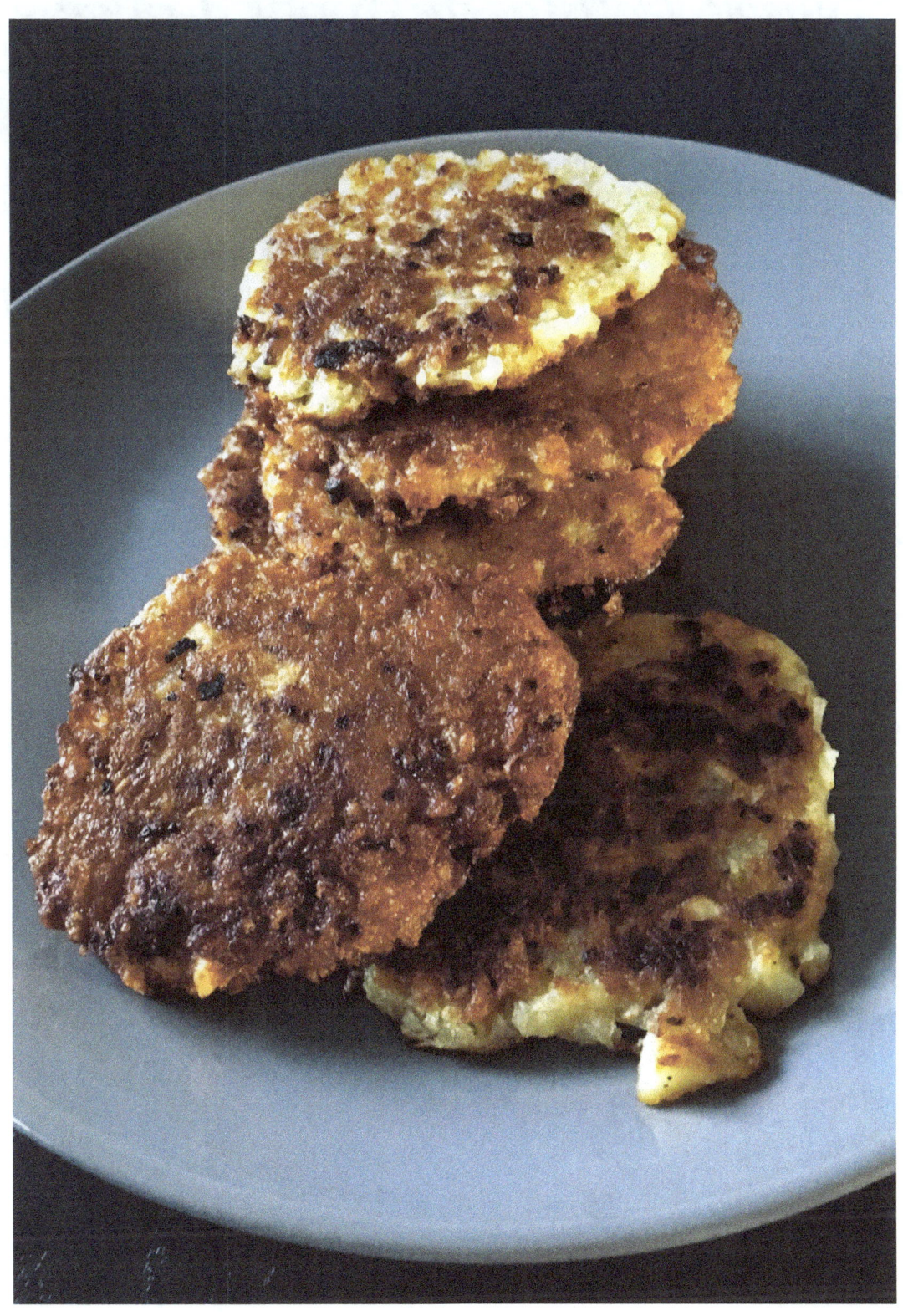

Sweet Potato & Apple Latkes

This fall festive latke combines everything we love about autumn. Apples are a nutrient and fiber-rich fruit that combines perfectly with the already luscious flavor of sweet potatoes. This recipe is a definite crowd pleaser!

MAKES 12 SERVINGS

INGREDIENTS

- 1 red apple, peeled and grated
- 2 medium sweet potatoes, peeled and grated
- 1 medium onion, chopped
- 2 egg whites
- ¾ cup all-purpose flour
- 1 tablespoon lemon juice
- ½ teaspoon ground cumin
- ½ teaspoon ground cinnamon
- 1 teaspoon olive oil

INSTRUCTIONS

1. In a large bowl, combine apple, sweet potatoes, and onion and mix thoroughly.
2. Beat egg whites and add to mixture.
3. Add flour, lemon juice, cumin, and cinnamon.
4. Coat a nonstick 12-inch skillet with olive oil and heat over medium heat.
5. Measure out 2 tablespoons of the mixture for each latke. Drop latkes into pan and cook until golden brown on both sides.

Crisp Potato Kugel

This recipe provides everything you love about a traditional potato kugel! The potatoes allow for a hearty consistency and a crisp outside that is both filling and satisfying.

MAKES 20 SERVINGS

INGREDIENTS

- 10 medium potatoes, grated
- 1 large onion, grated
- 4 egg whites
- 1 ½ teaspoons salt
- ⅛ teaspoon black pepper
- 2 tablespoons olive oil

INSTRUCTIONS

1. Preheat oven to 450°F.
2. Mix grated potatoes, onions, and egg whites. Season with salt and black pepper.
3. Pour olive oil into an 8 x 11-inch baking dish. Place in oven until hot. Pour heated oil into potato mixture. Using a paper towel, wipe out rest of oil from pan, making sure to coat the bottom and sides of dish.
4. Pour potato mixture into pan and bake for 45 minutes to 1 hour on the top shelf.

Carrot Kugel

What's not to love about a carrot cake turned kugel? Aside from the sweet, decadent taste, this kugel provides a burst of vitamin A and dietary fiber from the carrots. As if it can't get any better, this kugel is fluffy and soft, reminiscent of a soufflé.

MAKES 9 SERVINGS

INGREDIENTS

- 12 medium carrots, sliced
- 1 tablespoon low fat margarine
- 1 whole egg
- 3 egg whites
- ¼ cup sugar
- ½ cup all-purpose flour
- ½ teaspoon salt
- 2 teaspoons baking powder
- 1 tablespoon hot water

INSTRUCTIONS

1. Preheat oven to 350°F. Prepare an 8 x 8-inch baking dish with nonstick spray and set aside.
2. Steam carrots until soft. Add margarine and mash well.
3. Beat egg whites and add to carrot mixture.
4. Blend in sugar, flour, salt, baking powder, and hot water to mixture.
5. Add mixture to prepared pan and bake for approximately 1 hour.

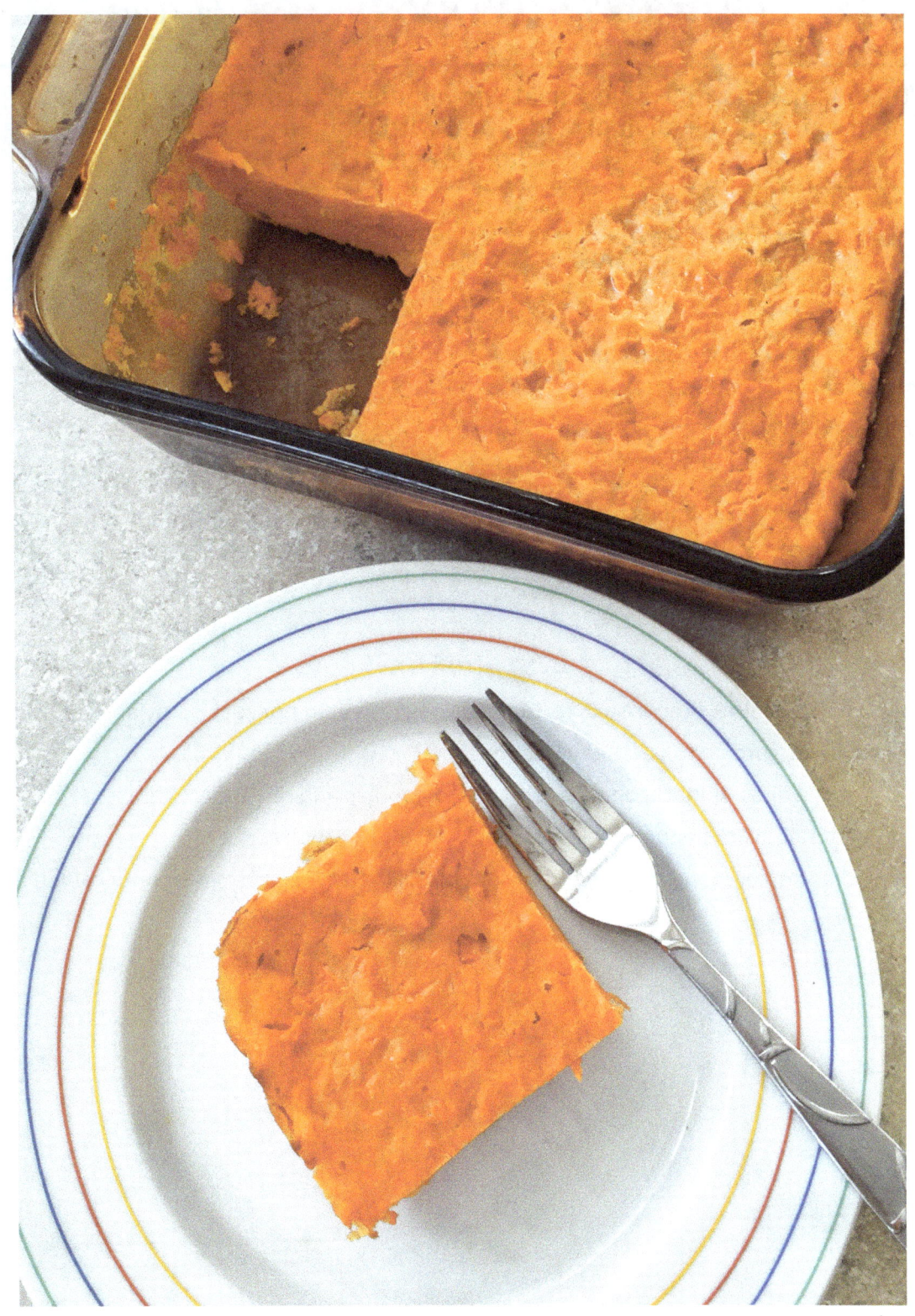

Spinach Noodle Kugel

This kugel is made with whole wheat egg noodles to provide extra fiber. With the addition of spinach, this dish provides you with a quality serving of vegetables and whole grains!

MAKES 16 SERVINGS

INGREDIENTS

- 1 (12-ounce) package uncooked medium whole wheat egg noodles
- 1 whole egg
- 2 egg whites
- 1 (10-ounce) box frozen spinach, thawed and strained
- 2 tablespoons light mayonnaise
- ½ teaspoon salt
- ½ teaspoon black pepper
- 1 teaspoon garlic powder
- 1 teaspoon onion powder

INSTRUCTIONS

1. Preheat oven to 350°F. Prepare a 9 x 13-inch baking dish with nonstick spray and set aside.
2. Cook noodles according to package directions.
3. Add egg, egg whites, spinach, and mayonnaise to noodles and mix thoroughly.
4. Season with salt, black pepper, garlic powder, and onion powder.
5. Pour noodles into prepared pan and bake for approximately 45 minutes or until golden brown.

Pineapple Kugel

Pineapple is the ultimate dessert fruit and provides this dish with a sweet island twist. Whether it's with a meal, as a dessert, during the holidays, or in the summer, this pineapple kugel will never fail to satisfy!

MAKES 9 SERVINGS

INGREDIENTS

- 1 (20-ounce) can crushed pineapple
- 2 whole eggs
- 4 egg whites
- ½ cup all-purpose flour
- ½ cup unsweetened applesauce
- ½ teaspoon baking powder
- 1 teaspoon vanilla extract
- ½ cup sugar
- Ground cinnamon, for garnish

INSTRUCTIONS

1. Preheat oven to 350°F. Prepare an 8 x 8-inch baking dish with nonstick spray and set aside.
2. Pour crushed pineapple into a mixing bowl.
3. Beat eggs and egg whites and add to pineapple.
4. Add flour, applesauce, baking powder, vanilla extract and sugar. Mix well.
5. Pour mixture into prepared pan. Bake for 40-45 minutes.
6. Sprinkle with cinnamon.

Intuitive Eating Wisdom

Intuitive Eating Principle 4:
Challenge the Food Police

It's time to challenge your negative thoughts about food. Shut out the notion that there are "good" versus "bad" foods and that you're "good" or "bad" for eating certain foods. Turn off the voice that you have picked up over the years that is reciting diet rules and shouting negative barbs at you. It will take time to turn down the noise until it's finally quiet. Transforming these negative voices into an ally within yourself is essential to intuitive eating.

Poultry & Meat

IN THIS CHAPTER

145 | Crispy Baked Chicken

146 | Versatile Chicken Breast

147 | Chicken Breast Toppers

149 | Chicken Scallopine with Marsala

150 | Italian Turkey Sauté

152 | Hawaiian Turkey Salad

153 | Kale-Stuffed Chicken Roll

154 | Balsamic Lemon Chicken

156 | Rosemary Chicken & White Bean Stew

157 | Beef & Asparagus Stir-Fry

158 | Bright Lemon Chicken

160 | Turkey & Apple Wrap

161 | Turkey & Mixed Bean Chili

162 | Orange Grilled Chicken Salad

164 | Home-Style Chicken Packets

Poultry & Meat

IN THIS CHAPTER

165 | Mediterranean Chicken & Rice Casserole

166 | Pomegranate-Orange Glazed Turkey

168 | Sweet Curried Chicken

169 | Cherry & Apricot Turkey Casserole

170 | Chicken & Broccoli Stir-Fry

172 | Marinated Beef Kebabs

173 | Tasty Chicken Sliders

174 | Beef Goulash

176 | Chicken Pot Pie

178 | Chicken Paprikash

Crispy Baked Chicken

If you're craving a hassle-free version of fried chicken, this recipe is for you. This baked chicken brings you all the crispiness you are looking for and is easy to prepare. Add corn on the cob and coleslaw for a satisfying meal.

MAKES 6 SERVINGS

INGREDIENTS

- 6 boneless chicken breasts (approximately 1 ½ pounds)
- 3 tablespoons Dijon mustard
- ½ cup plain bread crumbs
- ½ cup crushed corn flakes
- ½ teaspoon marjoram
- ¼ teaspoon sage
- ¼ teaspoon black pepper

INSTRUCTIONS

1. Preheat oven to 350°F.
2. Brush top of chicken with 2 tablespoons Dijon mustard.
3. Combine remaining tablespoon of Dijon mustard with bread crumbs, corn flake crumbs, marjoram, sage, and black pepper.
4. Pat mixture onto chicken and bake 30-40 minutes.

Versatile Chicken Breast

This chicken breast is just that – versatile! It is an easy to make chicken dish and a great basic recipe to have in your recipe box. Choose from three delicious toppers on the following pages to give additional flavor and added nutrients to your dish.

MAKES 4 SERVINGS

INGREDIENTS

- 4 boneless chicken breasts (approximately 1 pound)
- ½ teaspoon salt
- ¼ teaspoon black pepper
- 1 tablespoon lemon juice
- 1 tablespoon dry white wine

INSTRUCTIONS

1. Preheat oven to 350°F.
2. Coat a baking dish with nonstick cooking spray. Arrange chicken breasts in dish.
3. Sprinkle with salt and black pepper; drizzle with lemon juice and wine.
4. Cover tightly and bake until chicken is white all the way through and juices run clear, approximately 20-25 minutes.

Chicken Breast Toppers

Chicken is a great source of lean protein and can be enjoyed with a variety of flavors. Try one of these toppers the next time you prepare baked chicken cutlets to bring a tasty flavor and vibrant color to your chicken dish each night of the week!

Asian Chicken Topper

MAKES 6 SERVINGS

INGREDIENTS

- 2 teaspoons olive oil
- 8-ounces sliced fresh mushrooms
- 1 bunch scallions, sliced
- 1 pound asparagus, cut into 1-inch pieces
- 1 ½ teaspoons low sodium soy sauce
- 1 teaspoon sesame oil

INSTRUCTIONS

1. In a skillet, heat olive oil over medium-high heat.
2. Add sliced mushrooms and scallions. Sauté for 5 minutes.
3. Add asparagus, soy sauce, and sesame oil. Cook and stir until asparagus are crisp tender, approximately 3 minutes.
4. Place Asian Topper over chicken.

Cabbage-Apple Chicken Topper

MAKES 6 SERVINGS

INGREDIENTS

- 1 teaspoon olive oil
- 1 (8-ounce) package of coleslaw mix
- 1 medium apple, sliced
- 1 teaspoon sugar
- 1 tablespoon + ½ teaspoon apple cider vinegar

INSTRUCTIONS

1. In a skillet, heat olive oil over medium-high heat.
2. Add coleslaw mix, apple, sugar, and apple cider vinegar. Cook until vegetables are tender, about 10 minutes.
3. Place Cabbage-Apple Topper over chicken.

Colored Pepper Chicken Topper

MAKES 6 SERVINGS

INGREDIENTS

- 1 tablespoon olive oil
- 1 medium onion, sliced
- 1 medium red bell pepper, sliced
- 1 medium green bell pepper, sliced
- 1 clove garlic, minced

INSTRUCTIONS

1. In a skillet, heat olive oil over medium-high heat.
2. Add onion, red pepper, green pepper, and garlic. Cook and stir until vegetables are tender, about 10 minutes.
3. Place Colored Pepper Topper over chicken.

Chicken Scallopine with Marsala

This is a true family favorite. Mushrooms add texture and a boost of nutrients, while corn starch thickens the sauce, making it creamy and delightful. Try this dish over whole wheat fettuccini for dinner tonight.

MAKES 5 SERVINGS

INGREDIENTS

- ¼ pound thinly sliced fresh mushrooms
- 1 ½ teaspoons lemon juice
- 2 tablespoons olive oil
- 2 tablespoons corn starch
- ⅛ teaspoon black pepper
- 1 pound boneless chicken breasts
- 2 tablespoons hot water
- ¼ cup dry Marsala wine
- 1 clove garlic, finely chopped
- Chopped fresh parsley, for garnish

INSTRUCTIONS

1. In a nonstick skillet, sauté mushrooms with lemon juice and olive oil. Remove mushrooms with slotted spoon and set aside. Leave liquid in pan.
2. Combine corn starch and black pepper in plastic zip bag. Add chicken and shake until coated.
3. In the skillet from the mushrooms, brown the coated chicken over medium-high heat, approximately 2-3 minutes per side.
4. In a separate bowl, combine water, wine, garlic, and sautéed mushrooms. Add mixture to skillet.
5. Continue cooking in sauce until chicken is cooked through. Garnish with parsley.

Italian Turkey Sauté

Trade in typical red meat for lean turkey in this Italian-style sauté that combines tomatoes, red wine, oregano, and basil. It is a satisfying, easy-to-follow recipe that works as a healthy alternative to other Italian dishes.

MAKES 4 SERVINGS

INGREDIENTS

- ½ cup diced onion
- 2 teaspoons olive oil
- 2 cloves garlic, minced
- 1 ½ cups crushed tomatoes
- 2 tablespoons red wine
- 4 cups cooked, cubed boneless turkey breast
- 2 teaspoons chopped fresh oregano
- 2 tablespoons chopped fresh basil

INSTRUCTIONS

1. In a large skillet, sauté onion in olive oil over medium-high heat.
2. Add the garlic and continue to cook for 2 more minutes.
3. Add the crushed tomatoes and wine. Bring to a boil, then lower the heat and simmer for 10 minutes.
4. Add the cubed turkey, oregano, and basil.
5. Simmer for 5 minutes until heated through.

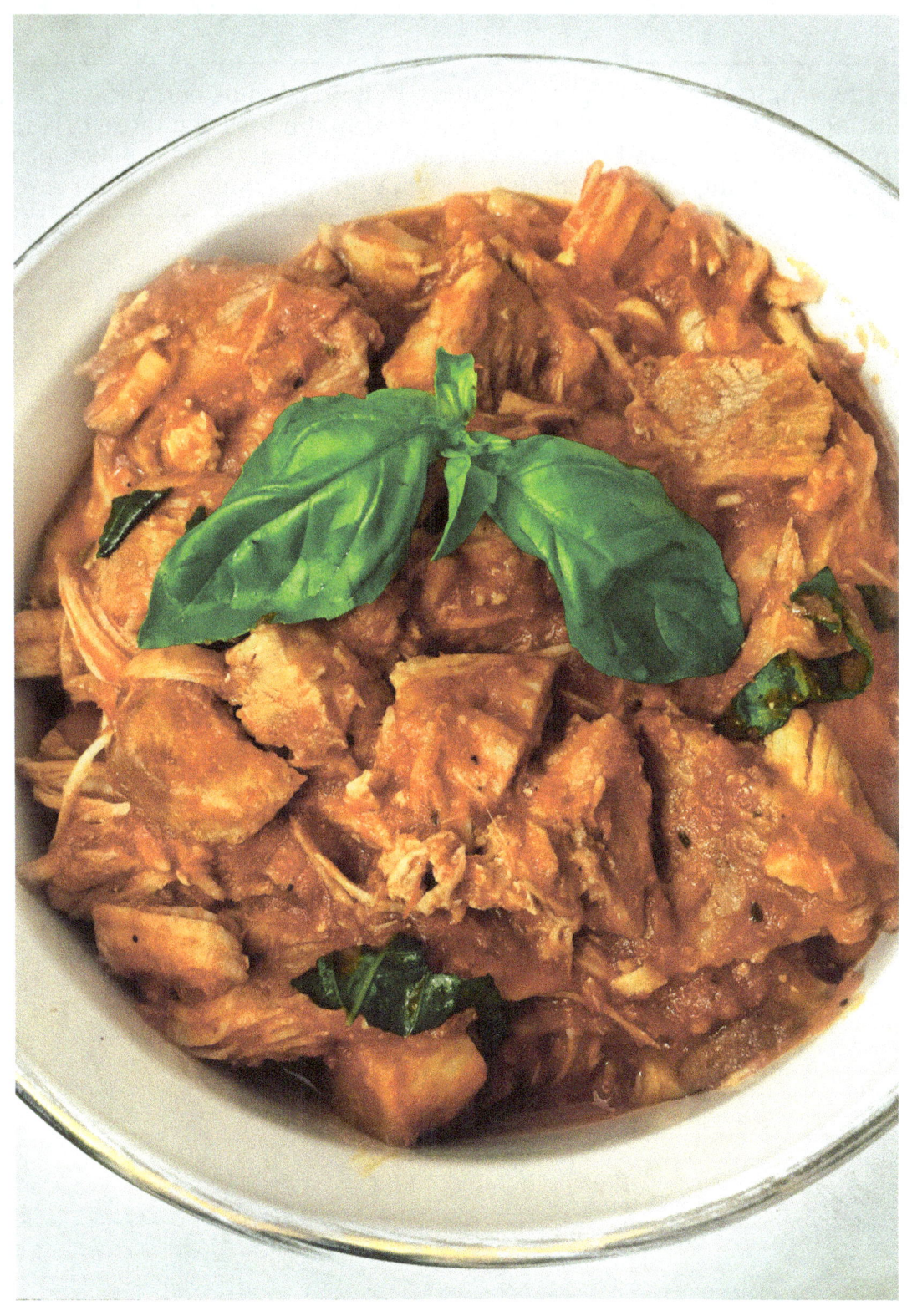

Hawaiian Turkey Salad

This healthy tropical salad is a great addition to any lunch or barbeque. Cinnamon and nutmeg give just the right amount of spice that adds even more of a flavor kick to the sweet fruits and crunchy vegetables. With turkey as the lean protein, this salad is filling and will surely have your guests coming back for more.

MAKES 8 SERVINGS

INGREDIENTS

- 3 cups cooked and cubed boneless turkey breast
- 2 cups diced celery
- 1 small onion, diced
- 1 cup diced Granny Smith apples
- ½ cup pineapple chunks in juice, drained
- ½ cup sliced grapes
- 3 tablespoons light mayonnaise
- ¼ teaspoon ground nutmeg
- ¼ teaspoon ground cinnamon
- ¼ teaspoon black pepper

INSTRUCTIONS

1. In a bowl, mix turkey, celery, onion, apples, pineapple, and grapes.
2. In a separate bowl, mix mayonnaise, nutmeg, cinnamon, and black pepper to make dressing.
3. Add dressing to turkey mixture and combine well.

Kale-Stuffed Chicken Roll

Kale is often touted as being the "Queen of Greens" as it is one of the most nutrient-dense vegetables. It packs in vitamins A, C, and K, plus calcium and potassium. This recipe is a great way to incorporate this leafy green into your next family meal.

MAKES 4 SERVINGS

INGREDIENTS

- 4 boneless chicken breasts (approximately 1 pound)
- 1 medium head fresh broccoli, chopped
- ½ cup chopped shallots
- ½ cup shredded carrots
- 2 cloves garlic, minced
- 1 tablespoon olive oil
- ¾ cup low sodium chicken broth
- 2 cups packed chopped kale
- 2 tablespoons light mayonnaise
- 1 teaspoon Dijon mustard
- ½ cup seasoned bread crumbs

INSTRUCTIONS

1. Preheat oven to 400°F. Prepare a baking dish with nonstick spray.
2. Pound chicken with mallet until thin and set aside.
3. Sauté broccoli, shallots, carrots and garlic in olive oil. Stir in chicken broth and cook for about 5 minutes or until shallots are tender, stirring frequently.
4. Add kale and cook until wilted, continuing to stir.
5. Spread 3 tablespoons kale mixture evenly over flattened chicken breasts. Roll chicken and secure with toothpicks.
6. In a separate bowl, mix mayonnaise and Dijon mustard. Coat chicken with mixture; then roll in bread crumbs.
7. Place chicken seam side down, in prepared baking dish. Bake 25 minutes or until chicken is golden brown and no longer pink near center. Remove toothpicks before serving.

Balsamic Lemon Chicken

Looking for another way to prepare chicken for dinner tonight? This recipe is easy to make and provides a delicious flavor of balsamic vinegar and lemon. Most of the ingredients can be found right in your kitchen!

MAKES 6 SERVINGS

INGREDIENTS

- 4 tablespoons balsamic vinegar, divided
- 4 tablespoons lemon juice, divided
- ¼ teaspoon black pepper
- 1 teaspoon corn starch
- 6 boneless chicken breasts (approximately 1 ½ pounds)
- 1 clove garlic, pressed
- 1 tablespoon chopped rosemary
- 1 teaspoon oregano
- 1 lemon, sliced

INSTRUCTIONS

1. In a bowl, combine 2 tablespoons of balsamic vinegar, 2 tablespoons of lemon juice, black pepper, and corn starch.
2. Add chicken to bowl and cover with marinade. Place in the refrigerator for 30 minutes.
3. Heat a nonstick skillet over medium heat until hot. Add marinated chicken cook 5 minutes. Turn chicken over.
4. Add remaining 2 tablespoons balsamic vinegar and 2 tablespoons lemon juice. Add the garlic, rosemary, oregano, and lemon wedges.
5. Cook another 6 minutes, or until chicken is cooked through and sauce slightly thickens.

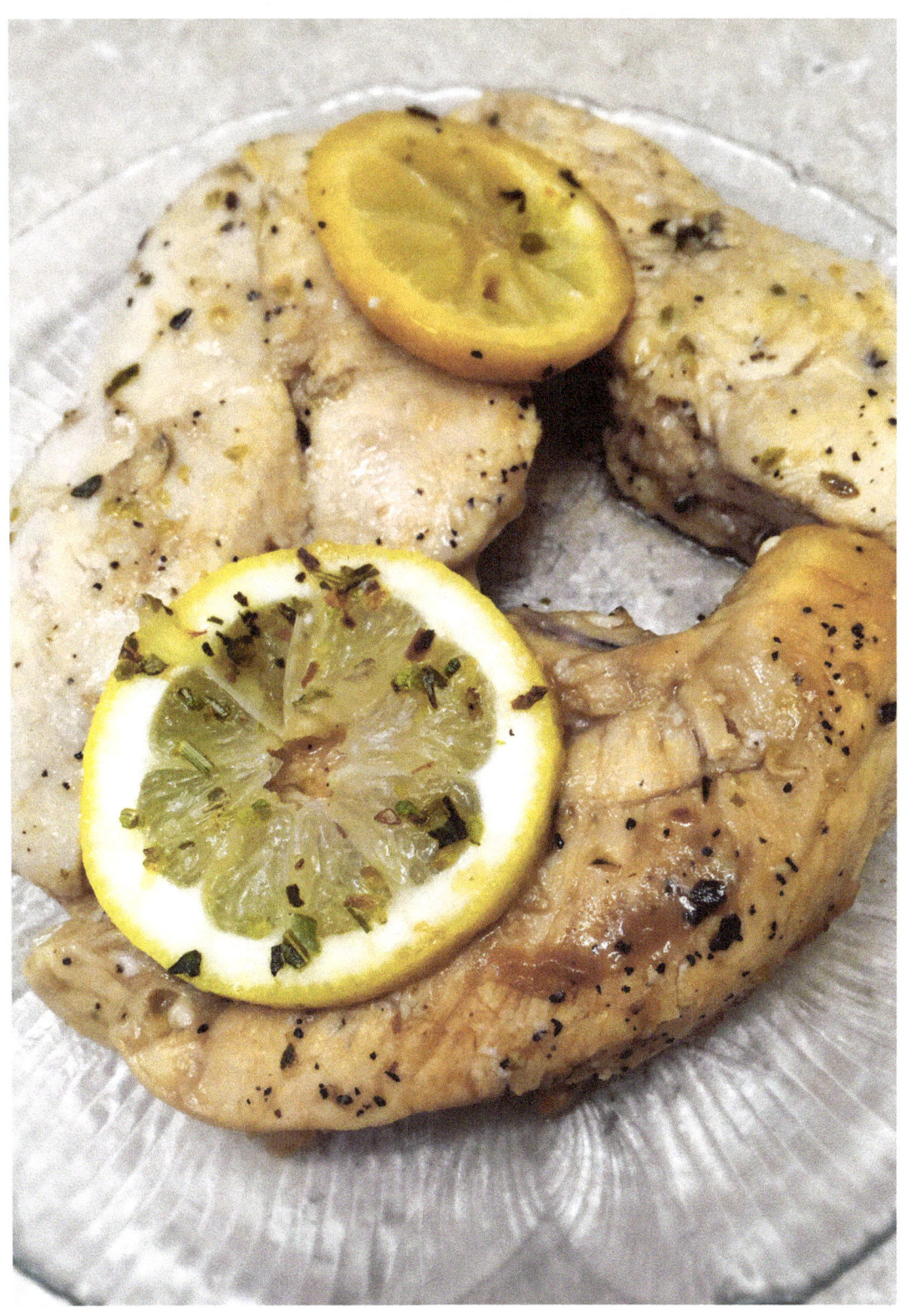

Rosemary Chicken
& White Bean Stew

This stew combines the rich flavors of eggplant, tomatoes, and chicken. Enjoy the addition of white beans for added texture and fiber. Use a piece of whole grain baguette to dip in and enjoy this meal until the very last bite.

MAKES 5 SERVINGS

INGREDIENTS

- 1 tablespoon olive oil
- 1 medium eggplant, diced
- 2 large stalks celery, chopped
- 1 teaspoon dried rosemary
- ½ teaspoon black pepper
- 1 pound boneless chicken breasts, cut into ¾-inch pieces
- 1 cup low sodium chicken broth
- 1 cup tomato sauce
- 1 (14-ounce) can stewed tomatoes
- 1 (15-ounce) can cannellini beans, drained and rinsed

INSTRUCTIONS

1. Heat oil in large saucepan over medium heat. Sauté eggplant and celery for 5 minutes, stirring occasionally.
2. Sprinkle rosemary and black pepper over chicken and add to saucepan. Cook for 2 minutes on each side.
3. Add chicken broth, tomato sauce, and stewed tomatoes and bring to a boil. Cover and simmer for 10 minutes.
4. Stir in beans and continue to simmer uncovered for 15 minutes or until chicken is cooked through.

Beef & Asparagus Stir-Fry

This is a quick meal that combines crisp vegetables and tender marinated beef. The variety of textures, colors, and flavors makes it a well-dressed dish with flare! Serve over a bed of steamed brown rice for a complete meal.

MAKES 6 SERVINGS

INGREDIENTS

- 1 teaspoon low sodium soy sauce
- 2 teaspoons ginger
- 2 cloves garlic, chopped
- 1 pound beef tenderloin, cubed
- 1 teaspoon olive oil
- 2 tablespoons water
- 10 asparagus spears, cut into 1-inch pieces
- 1 small yellow bell pepper, sliced
- 1 small onion, diced
- ⅓ cup low sodium chicken broth
- 1 teaspoon corn starch

INSTRUCTIONS

1. In a large mixing bowl, whisk together soy sauce, ginger, and garlic.
2. Coat beef tenderloin in marinade and refrigerate for 30 minutes.
3. In a large wok, sauté marinated beef in olive oil until no longer pink in center. Remove and set aside.
4. Add water, asparagus, yellow pepper, and onion to the wok. Cook for approximately 2 minutes.
5. In a separate pan, combine chicken broth and corn starch over low heat. Add to wok and stir until sauce is thickened and vegetables are crisp-tender.
6. Return beef to wok and heat for an additional 5 minutes.

Bright Lemon Chicken

This breaded chicken smothered in a slightly sweet lemon sauce is a crowd pleaser. Add roasted potatoes and vegetables for a nutrient-dense meal that everyone will enjoy.

MAKES 4 SERVINGS

INGREDIENTS

- 2 egg whites
- ¼ cup bread crumbs
- ¼ teaspoon black pepper
- 4 boneless chicken breasts (approximately 1 ¼ pounds)
- 2 tablespoons all-purpose flour
- 1 tablespoon olive oil
- ¾ cup low sodium chicken broth
- 4 teaspoons corn starch
- ¼ cup lemon juice
- 2 tablespoons brown sugar
- 1 tablespoon honey

INSTRUCTIONS

1. Place egg whites in a shallow dish.
2. In a separate dish, combine bread crumbs and black pepper.
3. Dust chicken with flour; dip into egg whites and roll in crumbs.
4. In a nonstick skillet, heat olive oil and cook chicken 5-8 minutes on each side or until chicken is cooked through. Transfer chicken to serving platter. Wipe skillet with paper towel.
5. In the same skillet, combine chicken broth and corn starch over low heat. Blend until smooth. Stir in lemon juice, brown sugar, and honey. Heat over medium-low heat and stir until broth boils and thickens.
6. Spoon sauce over chicken.

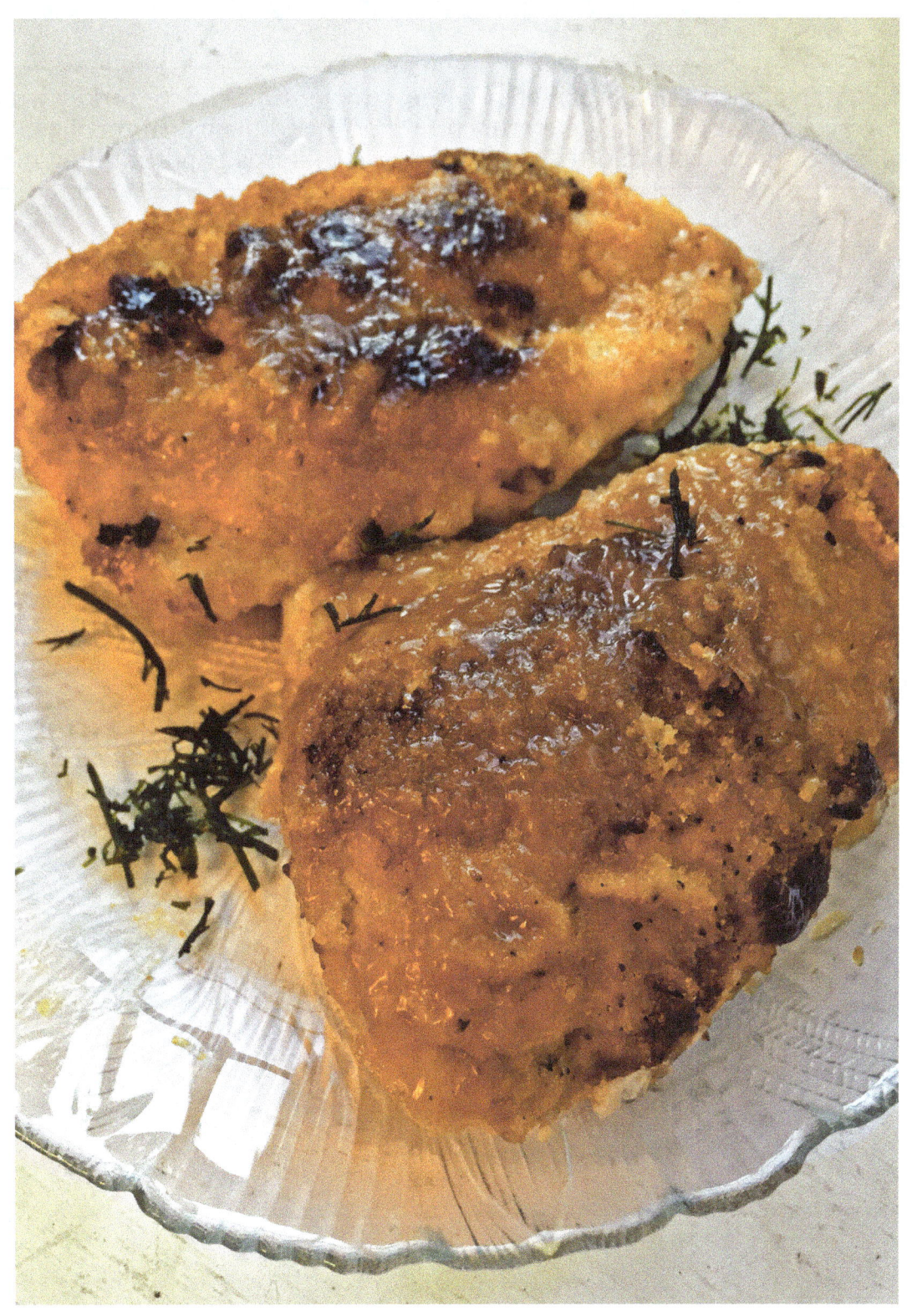

Turkey & Apple Wrap

Sliced crisp apples add a touch of sweetness to your lunchtime turkey wrap. Chopped celery and onions add a crunch to the soft whole wheat tortillas. This wrap has all the flavors and textures you desire in a fresh and fulfilling meal.

MAKES 4 SERVINGS

INGREDIENTS

- ¾ pound sliced turkey breast, cut into strips
- 1 medium apple, sliced
- ½ small red onion, chopped
- 1 stalk celery, chopped
- 2 cups fresh spinach leaves
- 1 tablespoon light mayonnaise
- 1 teaspoon Dijon mustard
- ½ tablespoon balsamic vinegar
- ⅛ teaspoon black pepper
- 4 whole wheat flour tortillas, heated

INSTRUCTIONS

1. In a large bowl, combine turkey, apple, red onion, celery, and spinach.
2. In a separate bowl, mix mayonnaise, Dijon mustard, balsamic vinegar, and black pepper.
3. Spread mayonnaise mixture on each tortilla.
4. Spoon turkey mixture down center of each tortilla. Fold sides of each tortilla over filling and roll.

Turkey & Mixed Bean Chili

Treat your body to a meal complete with carbohydrate, fiber and protein with this flavorful chili recipe. Cocoa powder and coffee add a special touch which elevates this dish to a new level of taste. This is a unique alternative to beef chili that will leave you feeling satisfied.

MAKES 8 SERVINGS

INGREDIENTS

- 1 small onion, diced
- ½ medium green bell pepper, diced
- 1 tablespoon olive oil
- 1 (6-ounce) can tomato paste
- 1 (15-ounce) can diced tomatoes
- ¾ tablespoon chili powder
- ½ teaspoon black pepper
- 6 jalapeno pepper, sliced
- 1 teaspoon unsweetened cocoa powder
- ⅓ cup brewed coffee
- 1 (16-ounce) can black beans, with liquid
- 1 (16-ounce) can small red beans, drained and rinsed
- 1 cup low sodium vegetable broth
- 10-ounces cooked boneless turkey breast, diced

INSTRUCTIONS

1. In a large pot, sauté onion and green pepper in olive oil over medium heat until soft.
2. Stir in tomato paste, tomatoes, chili powder, black pepper, jalapeno peppers, cocoa powder, and coffee. Heat for 5 minutes.
3. Add beans, cover and simmer for 5 minutes over low heat.
4. Add broth and bring to a boil, then lower to a simmer.
5. Add turkey to pan and heat through.

Orange Grilled Chicken Salad

Oranges add a refreshing and sweet citrus flavor to your typical chicken salad, and the sweet dressing lightly coats the chicken to produce a nice glaze. No need to add anything extra - eat it plain or between two slices of whole grain bread.

MAKES 6 SERVINGS

INGREDIENTS

- ½ cup orange juice
- ½ cup white wine vinegar
- ¼ cup olive oil
- ¼ tablespoon garlic and herb seasoning
- 1 ½ tablespoons sugar
- 1 pound boneless chicken breasts
- 4 cups romaine lettuce
- 1 (11-ounce) can mandarin oranges, drained
- ½ cup chopped green beans
- ½ cup shredded carrots

INSTRUCTIONS

1. Whisk together orange juice, white wine vinegar, olive oil, garlic and herb seasoning, and sugar to make dressing.
2. Brush chicken with ½ cup of dressing. Set aside remaining dressing.
3. Grill chicken until fully cooked, turning and brushing occasionally with dressing. Cut chicken into strips.
4. In a separate bowl, combine lettuce, oranges, green beans, and carrots. Toss in chicken.
5. Drizzle remaining dressing over salad.

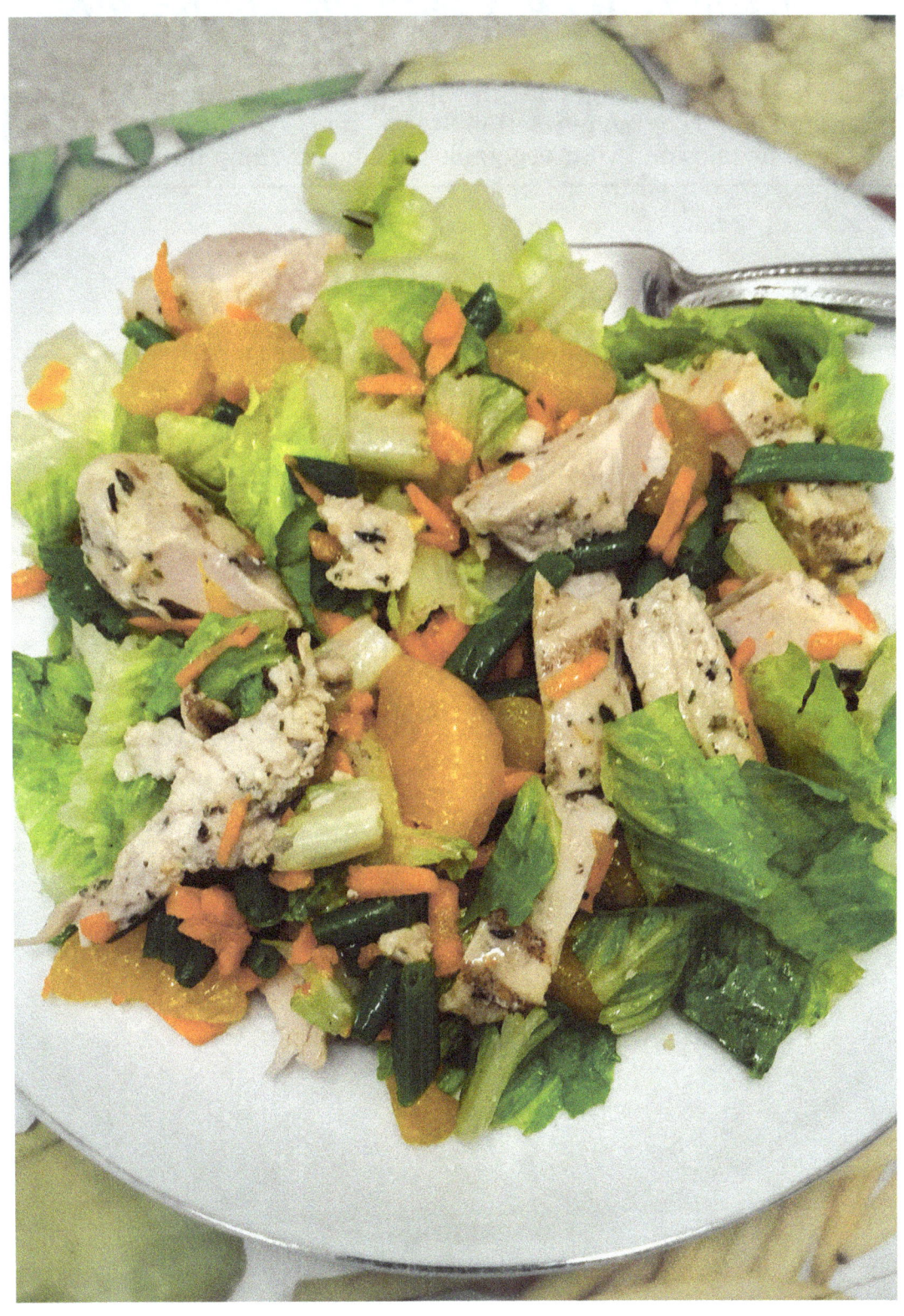

Home-Style Chicken Packets

Chicken and vegetables combined with Dijon mustard and spices are wrapped in aluminum foil and baked to perfection. It is a great way to ensure your chicken will be juicy and your vegetables will be anything but bland!

MAKES 4 SERVINGS

INGREDIENTS

- 4 boneless chicken breasts (approximately 1 pound)
- 4 teaspoons Dijon mustard
- 1 teaspoon dried basil
- 1 teaspoon paprika
- 2 medium carrots, sliced
- 2 cups sliced fresh mushrooms
- 2 medium zucchini, sliced

INSTRUCTIONS

1. Preheat oven to 450°F or preheat grill to medium-high.
2. Place each chicken breast on an individual sheet of aluminum foil.
3. Spread 1 teaspoon Dijon mustard over each piece of chicken; sprinkle with basil and paprika. Top with carrots, mushrooms, and zucchini.
4. Bring up sides of foil and double fold ends to form four packets, leaving room for heat circulation inside packets.
5. Bake 18-22 minutes in oven or grill 14-16 minutes on medium-high, covered.

Mediterranean Chicken
& Rice Casserole

This recipe has a variety of herbs and spices that gives this chicken dish a kick of flavor. It incorporates a perfect balance of whole grains, protein, and vegetables with flavors of oregano and paprika that will remind you of the Mediterranean.

MAKES 6 SERVINGS

INGREDIENTS

- 1 large onion, diced
- 1 cup chopped fresh mushrooms
- 2 cloves garlic, chopped
- 1 tablespoon olive oil
- 1 (10-ounce) box frozen chopped spinach, thawed
- ½ tablespoon oregano
- ½ tablespoon sage
- 1 tablespoon rosemary
- 1 teaspoon paprika
- 1 (6-ounce) can crushed tomatoes
- 1 cup uncooked quick cooking brown rice
- 2 teaspoons lemon juice
- 6 boneless chicken breasts, cut into thirds (approximately 1 ½ pounds)

INSTRUCTIONS

1. Preheat oven to 400°F.
2. In a nonstick skillet, sauté onion, mushrooms, and garlic in olive oil until tender.
3. Add spinach, oregano, sage, rosemary, and paprika and cook 5 minutes.
4. Add crushed tomatoes, brown rice, and lemon juice. Cook an additional 5 minutes.
5. Spread mixture in the bottom of a baking dish. Place chicken pieces on top.
6. Cook covered for 30 minutes in preheated oven until rice and chicken are cooked through. Remove cover and cook for an additional 5-6 minutes.

Pomegranate-Orange Glazed Turkey

This dish brings your taste buds right back to Thanksgiving! The sweet, tangy, mouthwatering flavor of the pomegranate-orange glaze compliment the roasted turkey breast and pairs with a side of your favorite roasted vegetables for a completely divine meal.

MAKES 16 SERVINGS

INGREDIENTS

- 3 ½ pounds boneless turkey breast
- Black pepper, to taste
- 1 tablespoon corn starch
- ½ cup pomegranate juice, divided
- 2 tablespoons honey
- 2 tablespoons balsamic vinegar
- ¼ cup low sodium chicken broth
- ¼ cup orange juice

INSTRUCTIONS

1. Preheat oven to 350°F.
2. Sprinkle both sides of turkey breast with black pepper and place on rack in shallow roasting pan. Cover and bake for 1-1 ¼ hours.
3. In a saucepan, combine corn starch with ¼ cup of pomegranate juice. Stir until corn starch dissolves and there is a smooth consistency.
4. Stir in remaining pomegranate juice, honey, balsamic vinegar, chicken broth, and orange juice. Bring to a boil and cook 1-2 minutes, until thickened.
5. Brush ½ of the glaze over the turkey breast; continue baking, uncovered, for 10 minutes. Repeat with remaining glaze and bake an additional 10 minutes.

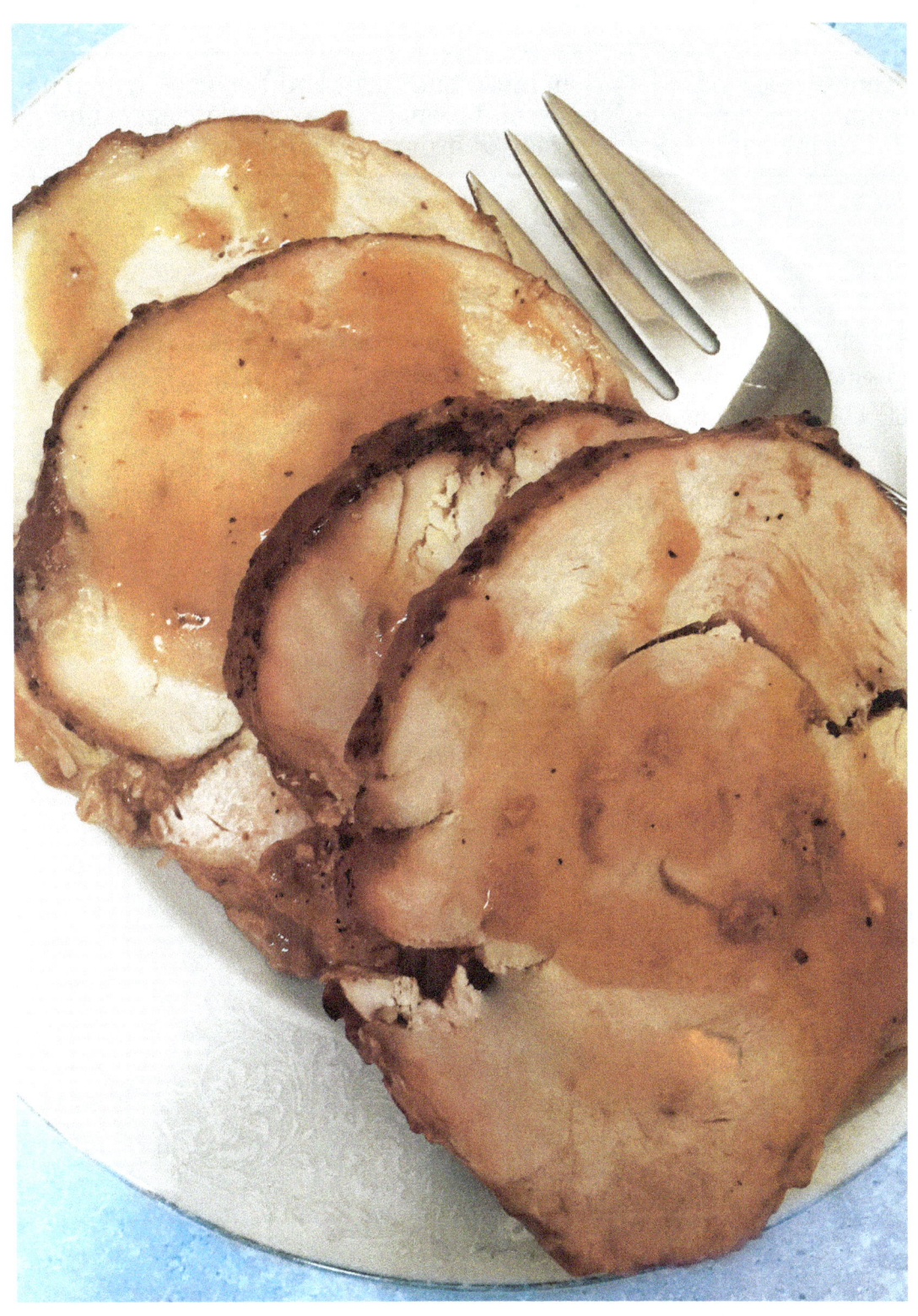

Sweet Curried Chicken

Turn your average baked chicken into a succulent and flavorful dish in no time. The combination of curry, honey, and orange will excite your taste buds. This recipe pairs well with a side of brown rice and roasted carrots.

MAKES 8 SERVINGS

INGREDIENTS

- 2 whole chickens, quartered and skinned (approximately 3½ pounds each)
- 2 tablespoons + 2 teaspoons honey, divided
- 2 tablespoons Dijon mustard
- 2 tablespoons low sodium chicken broth
- ¼ cup light mayonnaise
- 1 teaspoon curry powder
- 1 navel orange, chopped
- 5 cloves garlic, chopped

INSTRUCTIONS

1. Preheat oven to 350°F.
2. Place chicken in roasting pan.
3. In a small bowl, whisk 2 tablespoons honey, Dijon mustard, chicken broth, mayonnaise, and curry powder.
4. Brush mixture onto chicken and top with orange and garlic.
5. Bake uncovered for approximately 1 ¼ hours.
6. Remove chicken from oven and drizzle with 2 teaspoons honey. Return to oven and cook for an additional 2 minutes or until golden brown.

Cherry & Apricot Turkey Casserole

This casserole has the perfect combination of flavors and nutrients. The dried apricots and cherries add a sweet flavor to the savory turkey and brown rice while the sauce adds a rich and creamy texture to the dish.

MAKES 6 SERVINGS

INGREDIENTS

- 3 cups cooked brown rice
- ¼ cup dried apricots
- ¼ cup dried cherries
- 4 tablespoons low fat margarine
- 4 tablespoons all-purpose flour
- 1 cup plain soy milk
- 2 cups low sodium chicken broth
- 3 egg whites, beaten
- 1 medium onion, chopped
- 1 clove garlic, chopped
- ⅛ teaspoon black pepper
- ¼ teaspoon ground cumin
- 1 teaspoon dried parsley
- 4 cups shredded roasted turkey breast

INSTRUCTIONS

1. Preheat oven to 350°F. Prepare a casserole dish with nonstick spray.
2. In a large bowl, combine cooked rice with apricots and cherries.
3. In a saucepan, melt margarine. Add flour, soy milk, and chicken broth. Whisk until sauce thickens, approximately 4-6 minutes.
4. Mix in egg whites, onion, garlic, black pepper, cumin, and parsley.
5. Spread rice mixture in prepared casserole dish. Add turkey to the casserole dish and cover with sauce.
6. Bake for approximately 45 minutes.

Chicken & Broccoli Stir-Fry

Hold the phone! No need to order Chinese food tonight. This stir-fry made with ginger is reminiscent of traditional American-Chinese food, but made in your own kitchen! It has a fresh taste that your whole family will love.

MAKES 4 SERVINGS

INGREDIENTS

- 1 tablespoon tamari sauce
- 1 tablespoon corn starch
- 1 tablespoon white vinegar
- 1 tablespoon fresh ginger
- 1 clove garlic, minced
- ¼ teaspoon red pepper flakes
- 2 boneless chicken breasts, cubed (approximately 12-ounces)
- 2 teaspoons olive oil, divided
- 2 cups fresh broccoli florets, sliced diagonally ¼-inch thick
- 2 carrots, sliced diagonally ¼-inch thick
- 1 bunch scallions, sliced diagonally
- ¼ cup water

INSTRUCTIONS

1. Combine tamari sauce, corn starch, white vinegar, ginger, garlic, and red pepper flakes in bowl and mix well.
2. Coat chicken with mixture.
3. Heat wok or large skillet over high heat; add 1 teaspoon oil.
4. Add chicken and stir-fry for 4 minutes. Remove chicken and set aside.
5. Add remaining oil to wok. Add broccoli, carrots and scallions. Stir-fry 1 minute.
6. Add water and cook, scraping bottom of wok, until veggies are tender, 5-7 minutes.
7. Return chicken to wok and heat through.

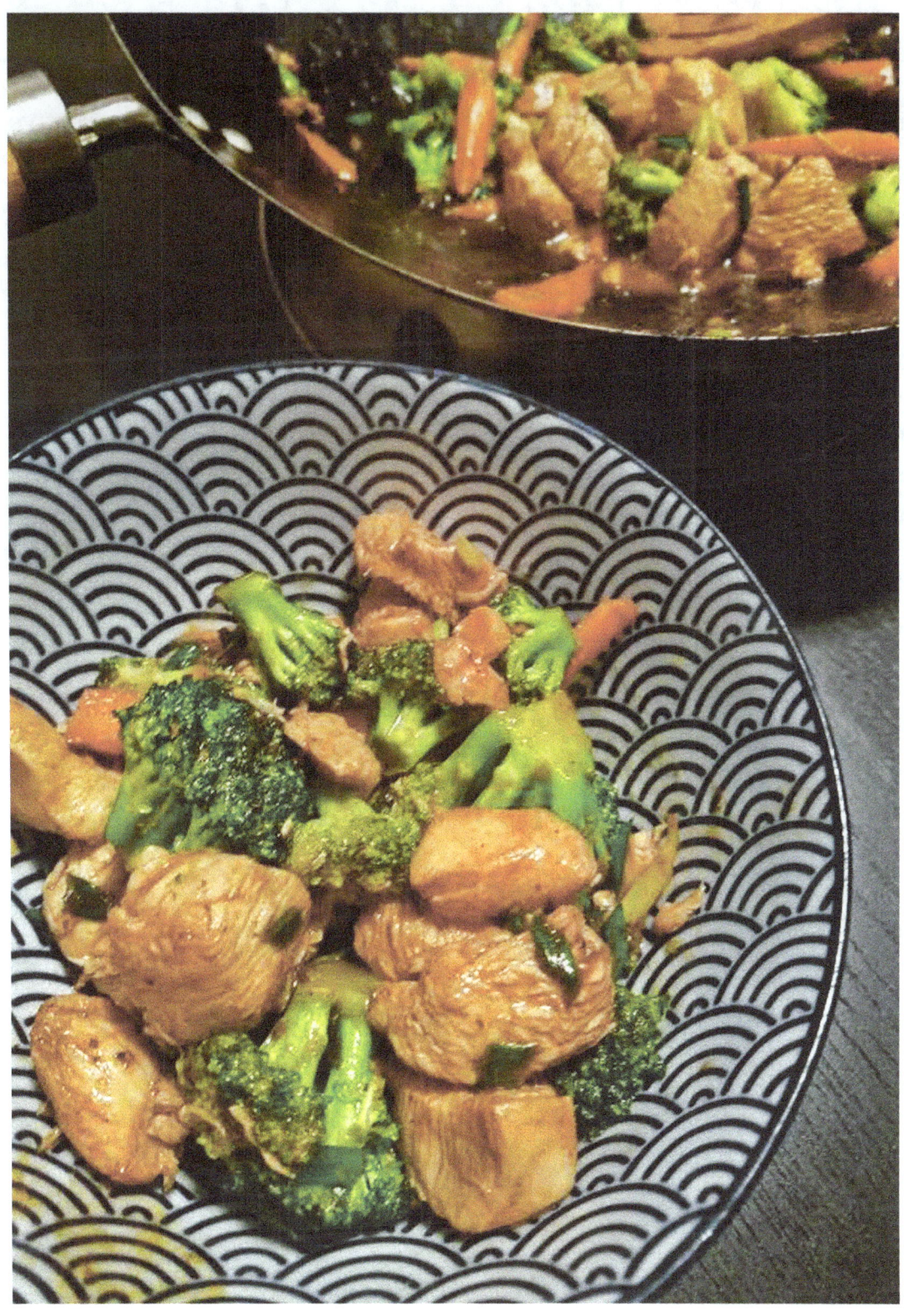

Marinated Beef Kebabs

These beef kebobs are a great addition to your barbeque menu. They pair well with a mixed vegetable medley and a side fruit salad. You can even get creative and switch up the veggies on the kebob.

MAKES 2 SERVINGS

MARINADE INGREDIENTS

- 2 tablespoons olive oil
- 1 clove garlic, chopped
- 2 tablespoons red wine vinegar
- 1 teaspoon lemon juice
- 1 tablespoon chopped dill

KEBOB INGREDIENTS

- 6-ounce brick roast, cut into 12 cubes
- 1 large onion, cut into cubes
- 18 cherry tomatoes
- 1 large green bell pepper, cut into large chunks
- 1 large yellow bell pepper, cut into large chunks

INSTRUCTIONS

1. In a small bowl, whisk together olive oil, garlic, red wine vinegar, lemon juice, and dill and set aside.
2. Mix brick roast, onion, tomatoes, and peppers in a bowl. Add marinade and toss well. Refrigerate for one hour.
3. Place beef and vegetables on 12-inch skewers, alternating each item.
4. Grill until beef is cooked through, about 10-12 minutes.

Tasty Chicken Sliders

These plump and juicy sliders are perfect for a day when you are in the mood for a not-so-typical burger. These are made with potatoes and onions for extra flavor and a great texture. Complete the sliders with a whole wheat bun and serve them at your next barbeque as an alternative to traditional hamburgers.

MAKES 10 SERVINGS

INGREDIENTS

- 16-ounces ground chicken breast
- 2 small potatoes, grated
- 1 large onion, grated
- 2 egg whites, beaten
- ½ teaspoon black pepper
- 1 teaspoon garlic powder
- 1 teaspoon onion powder
- 10 whole wheat mini burger buns (optional)

INSTRUCTIONS

1. In a large mixing bowl, combine ground chicken, potato, onion, and egg whites.
2. Season with black pepper, garlic powder, and onion powder.
3. Spray skillet with nonstick cooking spray and drop 2 tablespoons of mixture into pan.
4. Cook over medium-high heat until golden brown on both sides.
5. Place chicken sliders in mini burger buns or lay on a bed of greens.

Beef Goulash

The beef in this recipe is slow cooked to tender perfection and will melt in your mouth. Serve over whole-wheat noodles with a side of veggies for a complete meal.

MAKES 8 SERVINGS

INGREDIENTS

- 2 ½ pounds beef shoulder, cubed
- Salt, to taste
- Black pepper, to taste
- 2 teaspoons olive oil, divided
- 2 onions, chopped
- 2 tablespoons paprika
- 2 teaspoons caraway seeds
- ½ tablespoon dried thyme
- 1 ½ tablespoons dried marjoram
- ⅛ teaspoon black pepper
- 4 cups low sodium chicken broth, divided
- 3 tablespoons tomato paste
- 2 tablespoons balsamic vinegar
- 2 cloves garlic, chopped
- 1 tablespoon sugar
- 2 bay leaves

INSTRUCTIONS

1. Season beef cubes with salt and black pepper.
2. In a sauté pan, heat 1 teaspoon oil over high heat. Brown meat on all sides, approximately 8 minutes. Transfer beef to a large pot and set aside.
3. Add chopped onions to sauté pan with beef drippings. Over medium heat, add remaining oil and sauté for approximately 5 minutes. Add onions to the large pot with beef.
4. In the same sauté pan, toast paprika, caraway seeds, thyme, marjoram and black pepper over medium heat for approximately 3 minutes or until fragrant.
5. Stir in 1 cup chicken broth to deglaze the pan. Transfer to pot with beef and onions.
6. Add tomato paste, balsamic vinegar, garlic, sugar, and bay leaves to the pot with the beef. Pour in remaining 3 cups of chicken broth. Stir to combine. Bring to a boil, then reduce heat.
7. Simmer for approximately 2 hours, periodically testing meat for softness with a fork.

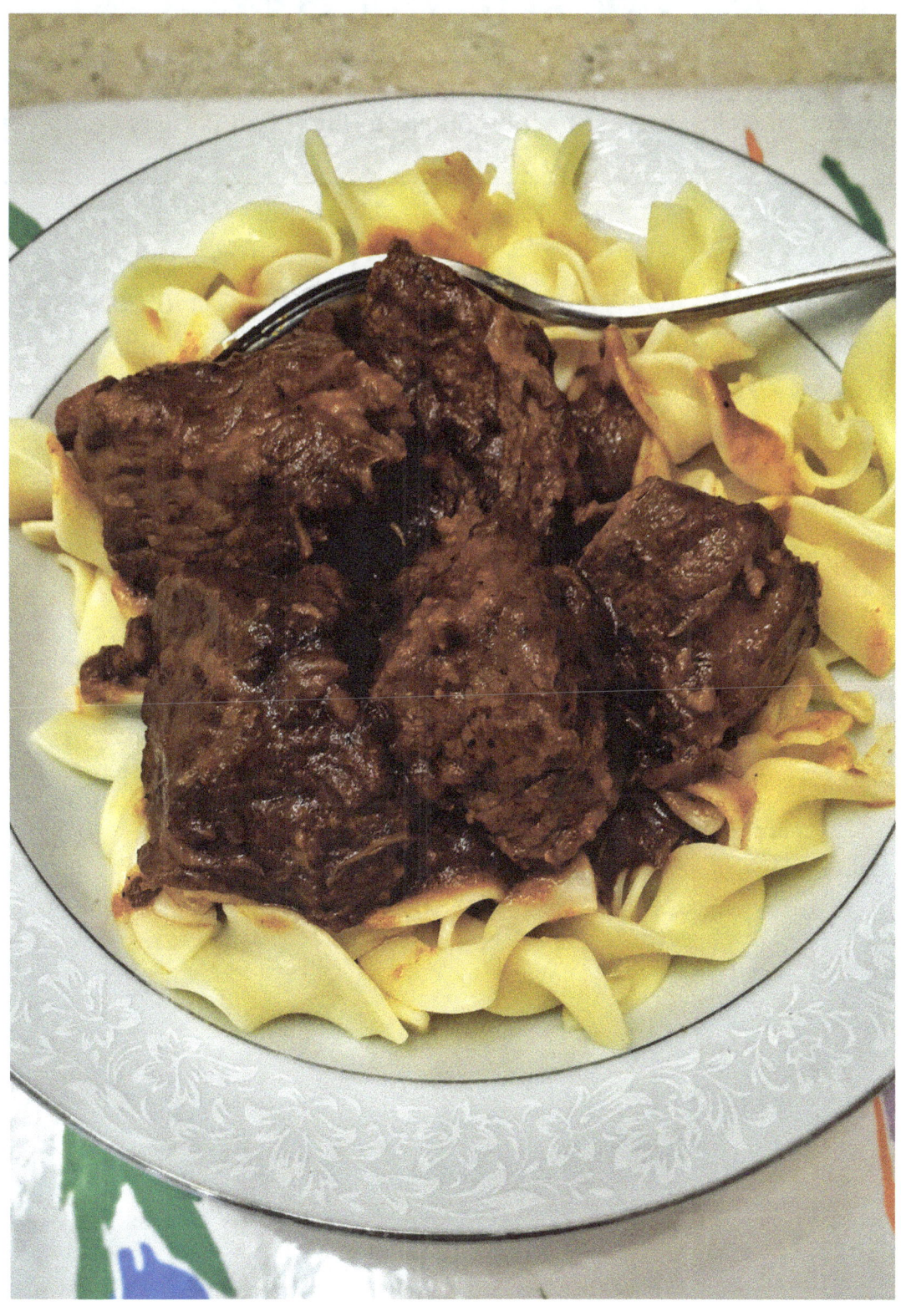

Chicken Pot Pie

There is nothing quite like this popular southern comfort food! Make your own flaky version of a classic crust to compliment a filling that is rich with flavor and nutrients.

MAKES 6 SERVINGS

FILLING INGREDIENTS

- 2 teaspoons olive oil
- 2 tablespoons + ½ cup low sodium chicken broth, divided
- 1 cup sliced fresh mushrooms
- ½ cup chopped green bell pepper
- ½ cup chopped red bell pepper
- 1 small onion, chopped
- 1 stalk celery, chopped
- 2 tablespoons all-purpose flour
- ½ cup plain soy milk
- 1 cup cooked chopped boneless chicken breasts
- 1 teaspoon chopped fresh parsley
- ¼ teaspoon black pepper

PIE CRUST INGREDIENTS

- ⅓ cup whole wheat flour
- ⅓ cup all-purpose flour
- ½ teaspoon salt
- 6 tablespoons olive oil
- ¼ cup plain soy milk

Poultry & Meat

INSTRUCTIONS

1. Preheat oven to 375°F.
2. In a saucepan, mix olive oil and 2 tablespoons chicken broth; heat over medium-heat.
3. Add mushrooms, green pepper, red pepper, onion, and celery. Cook until vegetables are fork-tender.
4. Mix in all-purpose flour and remaining chicken broth and cook until a thick consistency.
5. Reduce to low heat and slowly stir in soy milk.
6. Add in chicken, parsley, and black pepper.
7. Place chicken mixture in a 1 ½ quart baking dish and set aside.
8. In a large mixing bowl, combine whole wheat flour and all-purpose flour with salt.
9. In a separate bowl, mix together olive oil and soy milk. Mix into dry ingredients.
10. Form dough into a ball. Roll dough between sheets of wax paper to flatten to form a 5-6 inch "pancake".
11. Peel off the top sheet and place dough on top of chicken mixture in baking dish.
12. Trim and flute. Bake for approximately 30 minutes until top is golden and filling is bubbling.

Chicken Paprikash

Paprika is used in this recipe to add a mildly sweet pepper flavor. The onions absorb all of the great flavors of the tomatoes, garlic and seasonings. Serve over whole wheat egg noodles with a side of roasted zucchini to complete the dish.

MAKES 8 SERVINGS

INGREDIENTS

- 8 (4-ounce) boneless chicken breasts
- 4 tablespoons paprika
- ¼ teaspoon black pepper
- 3 cloves garlic, minced
- 1 medium onion, chopped
- 1 tablespoon olive oil
- 8 medium tomatoes, peeled and diced
- ½ cup water
- 1 tablespoon ketchup

INSTRUCTIONS

1. Season chicken breasts with paprika and black pepper.
2. In a skillet coated with nonstick spray, sauté garlic and onion in olive oil for 3-4 minutes.
3. Add chicken and cook on medium-heat for approximately 15 minutes.
4. In a separate saucepan, bring peeled tomatoes and water to a simmer. Add ketchup and heat through.
5. Add tomato sauce mixture to chicken and simmer another 15-20 minutes or until chicken is tender.

Intuitive Eating Wisdom

Intuitive Eating Principle 5: Respect Your Fullness

Eat with full consciousness so you can be aware of when you feel comfortably full. Observe the way your body communicates this to you by eating slowly and with attention to the sensations you're experiencing. When you feel you're full, respect this feeling, knowing you have full permission to eat this food again when you feel hungry.

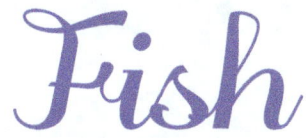

IN THIS CHAPTER
---

183 | Zesty Salmon Fillets

184 | Mahi-Mahi Tacos with Tropical Salsa

186 | Grilled Salmon with Honey Mustard Dill Sauce

187 | Tuna Noodle Casserole

188 | Bruschetta Baked Tilapia

190 | Mediterranean Tuna Pouches

191 | Moroccan Salmon

192 | Lemon Garlic Salmon

194 | Broiled Tilapia with Zesty Mandarin Orange Relish

195 | Lemon Pepper Halibut with Linguine

196 | Broiled Fish Fillets with Mustard

198 | Orange-Glazed Salmon

199 | Open-Faced Tuna Melt

200 | Vegetable & Fish Stir-Fry

201 | Tuna Boats

Zesty Salmon Fillets

Classic flavors are combined into a marinade that will wake up your taste buds. This tangy vinaigrette will add zest to your salmon and will certainly be a hit with your family!

MAKES 4 SERVINGS

INGREDIENTS

- 2 (4-ounce) salmon fillets
- 1 tablespoon light mayonnaise
- 2 tablespoons balsamic vinegar
- 2 tablespoons yellow mustard

INSTRUCTIONS

1. Broil salmon fillets for 5 minutes.
2. Mix together mayonnaise, balsamic vinegar, and mustard.
3. Spread mixture on top of each fillet and broil for another 5 minutes.

Mahi-Mahi Tacos
with Tropical Salsa

This dish will have you feeling like you are on vacation in the tropics! The delicate flavor of mahi-mahi is seasoned with chili powder and coriander and topped with cabbage and tropical salsa. Make this dish for a summer get-together and your family and friends will be very impressed!

MAKES 4 SERVINGS

TROPICAL SALSA INGREDIENTS

- 1 cup diced fresh strawberries
- ½ cup diced mango
- ¼ cup diced papaya
- ¼ cup diced pineapple
- ¼ cup diced green bell pepper
- 2 tablespoons diced red onion
- 2 tablespoons chopped scallions
- 2 tablespoons lime juice
- 1 tablespoon chopped fresh cilantro
- 1 ½ teaspoons rice vinegar
- Cayenne pepper, to taste

TACO INGREDIENTS

- 1 pound mahi-mahi, cut into eight pieces
- ¼ teaspoon black pepper
- ¼ teaspoon ground cumin
- ¼ teaspoon coriander
- ¼ teaspoon chili powder
- 8 (6-inch) whole grain corn tortillas
- 2 cups shredded cabbage

INSTRUCTIONS

1. Gently mix all salsa ingredients together and season with cayenne pepper to taste. Set aside.
2. Season mahi-mahi with black pepper, cumin, coriander, and chili powder. Place on grill and cook until fish is firm and reaches an internal temperature of at least 145°F.
3. In the meantime, warm the tortillas in the oven or on the grill.
4. Top each tortilla with equal amounts of fish, cabbage, and tropical salsa.

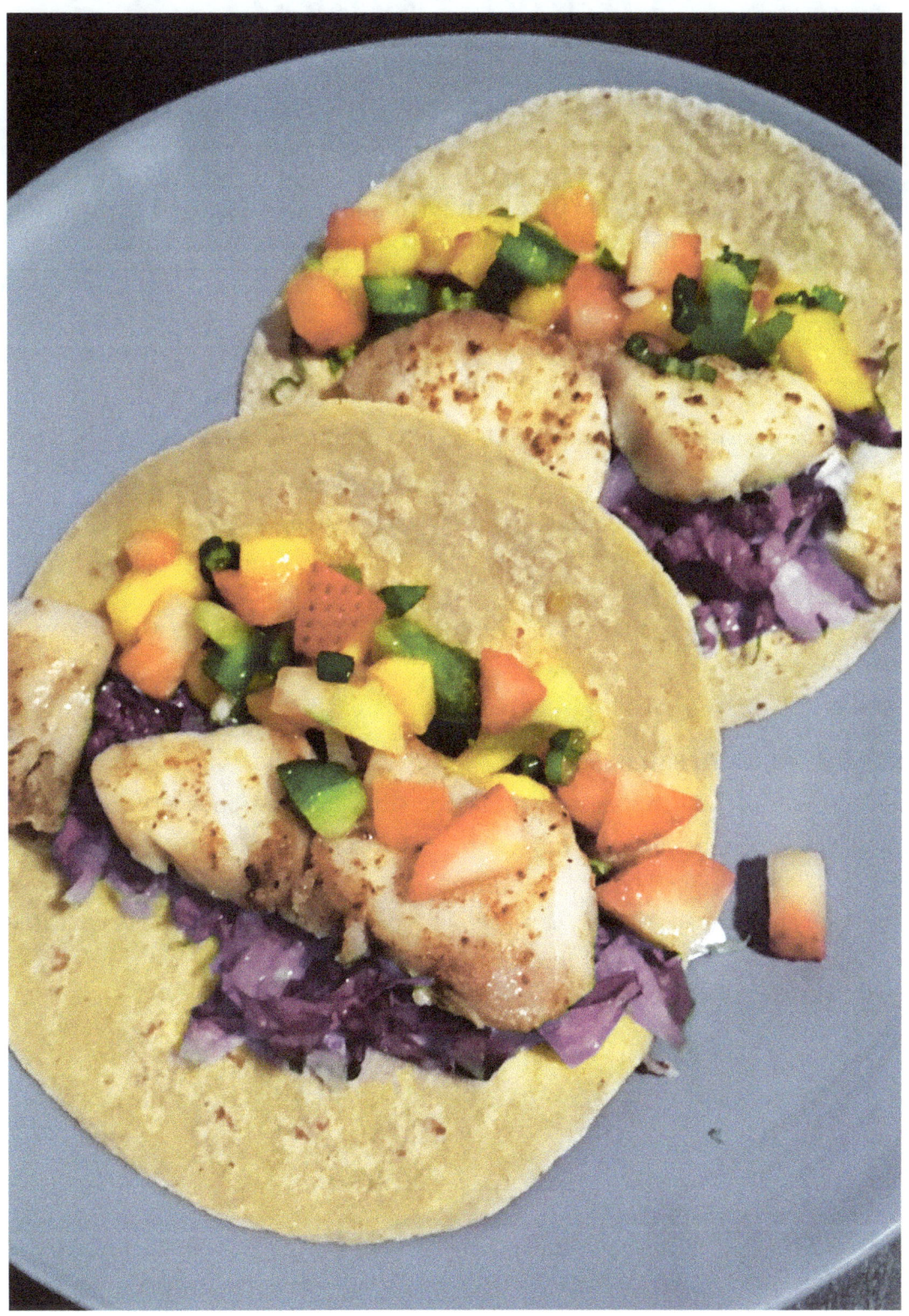

Grilled Salmon
with Honey Mustard Dill Sauce

The sweet flavor of honey and the mild spice of Dijon mustard compliment the distinct flavor of salmon. Pair this dish with a side of seasoned brown rice and enjoy the taste of eating out without leaving your home.

MAKES 4 SERVINGS

INGREDIENTS

- 4 (6-ounce) salmon steaks (approximately 1-inch thick)
- ½ teaspoon salt, divided
- ½ teaspoon black pepper, divided
- ½ cup plain nonfat yogurt
- 1 teaspoon honey
- ¾ tablespoon Dijon mustard
- ¼ cup chopped fresh dill
- 1 tablespoon minced scallions

INSTRUCTIONS

1. Prepare grill rack with nonstick spray.
2. Season both sides of salmon steak with ¼ teaspoon salt and ¼ teaspoon black pepper.
3. In a small bowl, combine yogurt, honey, Dijon mustard, dill, scallions, and remaining salt and pepper. Stir well and set aside.
4. Place salmon on prepared grill rack. Grill 6 minutes on each side or until fish flakes easily when tested with a fork.
5. Top with sauce to serve.

Fish

Tuna Noodle Casserole

Made with whole wheat egg noodles, tuna, cream sauce, and vegetables, this casserole has everything you desire from this classic comfort food dish! This is a quick recipe that tastes delicious and is easy to make with ingredients you may already have.

MAKES 4 SERVINGS

INGREDIENTS

- 1 cup sliced fresh mushrooms
- ½ cup chopped red bell pepper
- 2 tablespoons chopped onion
- 3 tablespoons butter
- 4 ½ tablespoons all-purpose flour
- 3 cups low fat milk
- 4 cups cooked whole wheat egg noodles
- 1 cup frozen green peas
- ¼ teaspoon salt
- ⅛ teaspoon black pepper
- 2 (6-ounce) cans tuna, in water, drained
- 2-ounces shredded low fat Cheddar cheese
- ¼ cup bread crumbs

INSTRUCTIONS

1. Preheat oven to 350°F.
2. Coat saucepan with nonstick spray; place over medium heat until hot. Add mushrooms, red pepper, and onion and sauté for 3 minutes or until crisp-tender. Remove from saucepan and set aside.
3. Heat butter in same saucepan over medium-low heat until melted. Add flour and cook 1 minute, stirring constantly with a wire whisk. Gradually add milk, stirring until thick and bubbly.
4. Stir in mushroom mixture, noodles, green peas, salt, black pepper, and tuna. Spoon into shallow 2-quart baking dish coated with nonstick spray. Top with cheese and bread crumbs.
5. Cover and bake for 20 minutes. Uncover and cook for an additional 10 minutes.

Bruschetta Baked Tilapia

The flavorful ingredients of the bruschetta are a delicious way to liven up the typical flavor of tilapia. Baking fish is a fool-proof method for preparing a quick and easy meal any time.

MAKE 4 SERVINGS

INGREDIENTS

- 1 teaspoon lemon juice
- 4 tilapia fillets (approximately 1 pound)
- ⅛ teaspoon black pepper
- 1 large tomato, diced
- 1 clove garlic, chopped
- 2 tablespoons chopped pitted ripe green olives
- 1 teaspoon onion powder
- ¼ teaspoon crushed red pepper (optional)
- 1 teaspoon chopped fresh parsley

INSTRUCTIONS

1. Preheat oven to 400°F. Prepare a baking dish with nonstick spray and set aside.
2. Drizzle lemon juice over tilapia. Season with black pepper and set aside.
3. To make bruschetta mixture, combine tomato, garlic, olives, onion powder, crushed red pepper, and parsley.
4. Place tilapia in prepared baking dish and top fish with bruschetta mixture.
5. Bake for approximately 15-20 minutes or until fish is flakes easily with a fork.

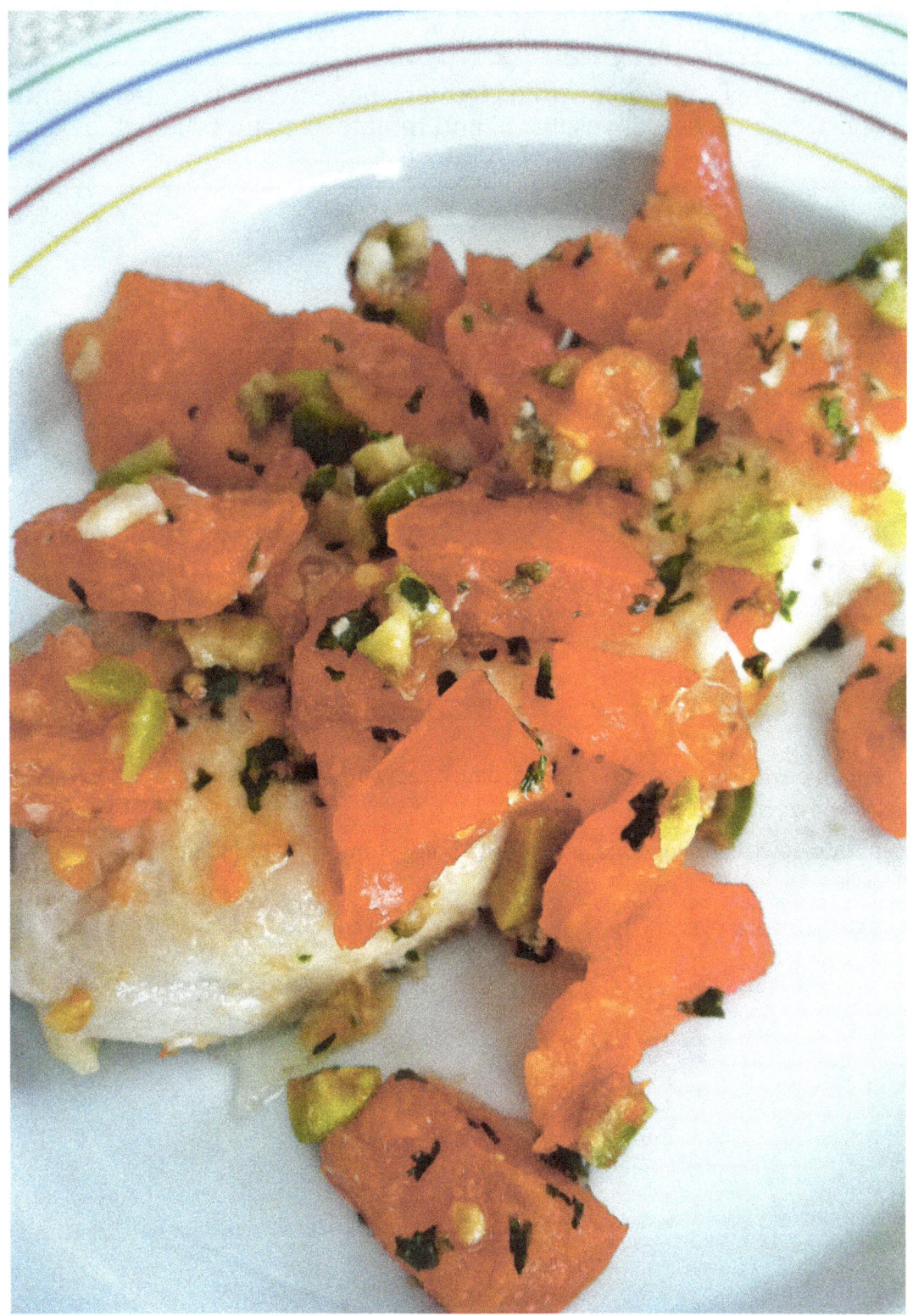

Mediterranean Tuna Pouches

Tune up your tuna sandwich with a Mediterranean twist! With ingredients like Greek yogurt, feta cheese, olives, basil, and tomatoes, plain tuna will be a memory from the past.

MAKES 6 SERVINGS

INGREDIENTS

- ½ cup plain nonfat Greek yogurt
- ½ cup red wine vinegar
- 2 tablespoons feta cheese
- ½ teaspoon dried oregano
- ½ teaspoon dried basil
- ¼ teaspoon onion powder
- 2 (6-ounce) cans tuna, in water, drained
- ½ cup jicama, cubed
- ½ small red onion, chopped
- 1 cup halved cherry tomatoes
- ½ cup diced red bell pepper
- ¼ cup diced olives (optional)
- 4 small whole wheat pita breads

INSTRUCTIONS

1. In a medium bowl, whisk together Greek yogurt, red wine vinegar, feta cheese, oregano, basil, and onion powder.
2. In a separate bowl, combine tuna, jicama, red onion, tomatoes, red pepper, and olives and gently mix.
3. Pour yogurt dressing over the tuna mixture and toss to coat. Refrigerate for 1 hour.
4. Spoon tuna mixture into pita pockets and serve.

Fish

Moroccan Salmon

The saffron, paprika, and cilantro elevate the flavors of this recipe to a whole new level of enjoyment! This dish is a great way to break free from your regular dinner routine and introduce your family to the tastes of Middle-Eastern cuisine. Serve with couscous for a more culturally authentic meal!

MAKES 8 SERVINGS

INGREDIENTS

- 1 medium green bell pepper, cut into julienne strips
- 1 medium red bell pepper, cut into julienne strips
- 1 medium yellow bell pepper, cut into julienne strips
- 2 medium plum tomatoes
- 2 jalapeno peppers, cut into julienne strips
- 2 pounds fresh fillet salmon, skinless, cut in 8 pieces
- 4 cloves garlic, chopped
- 2 teaspoons paprika
- 6 to 7 threads of saffron
- ¼ cup olive oil
- Juice of 1 lemon
- ¼ cup water
- ⅛ teaspoon salt
- ⅛ teaspoon black pepper
- ½ cup loosely packed cilantro

INSTRUCTIONS

1. Preheat oven to 350°F. Prepare a large baking dish with nonstick spray.
2. Place green, red, and yellow peppers, tomatoes, and jalapeno peppers on baking dish and top with salmon.
3. In small mixing bowl, combine garlic, paprika, saffron, olive oil, lemon juice, water, salt, and black pepper.
4. Pour mixture over salmon. Cover with foil and bake for 45 minutes, basting once or twice during cooking.
5. Add cilantro during last 5 minutes of cooking.

Lemon Garlic Salmon

Be your own professional chef with this simple yet elegant meal. The hint of garlic and lemon pepper brings this fish to life in a quick and delicious way!

MAKES 2 SERVINGS

INGREDIENTS

- 1 tablespoon olive oil
- 1 clove garlic, minced
- 2 (6-ounce) salmon fillets
- 1 teaspoon lemon pepper
- 1 teaspoon lemon juice

INSTRUCTIONS

1. Heat olive oil in a nonstick skillet over medium-high heat. Stir in minced garlic.
2. Season salmon fillets on both sides with lemon pepper.
3. Place the fillets in the skillet to cook. Flip the fillets midway to brown on each side. Cook until fillets flake when tested with a fork.
4. Sprinkle with lemon juice and serve.

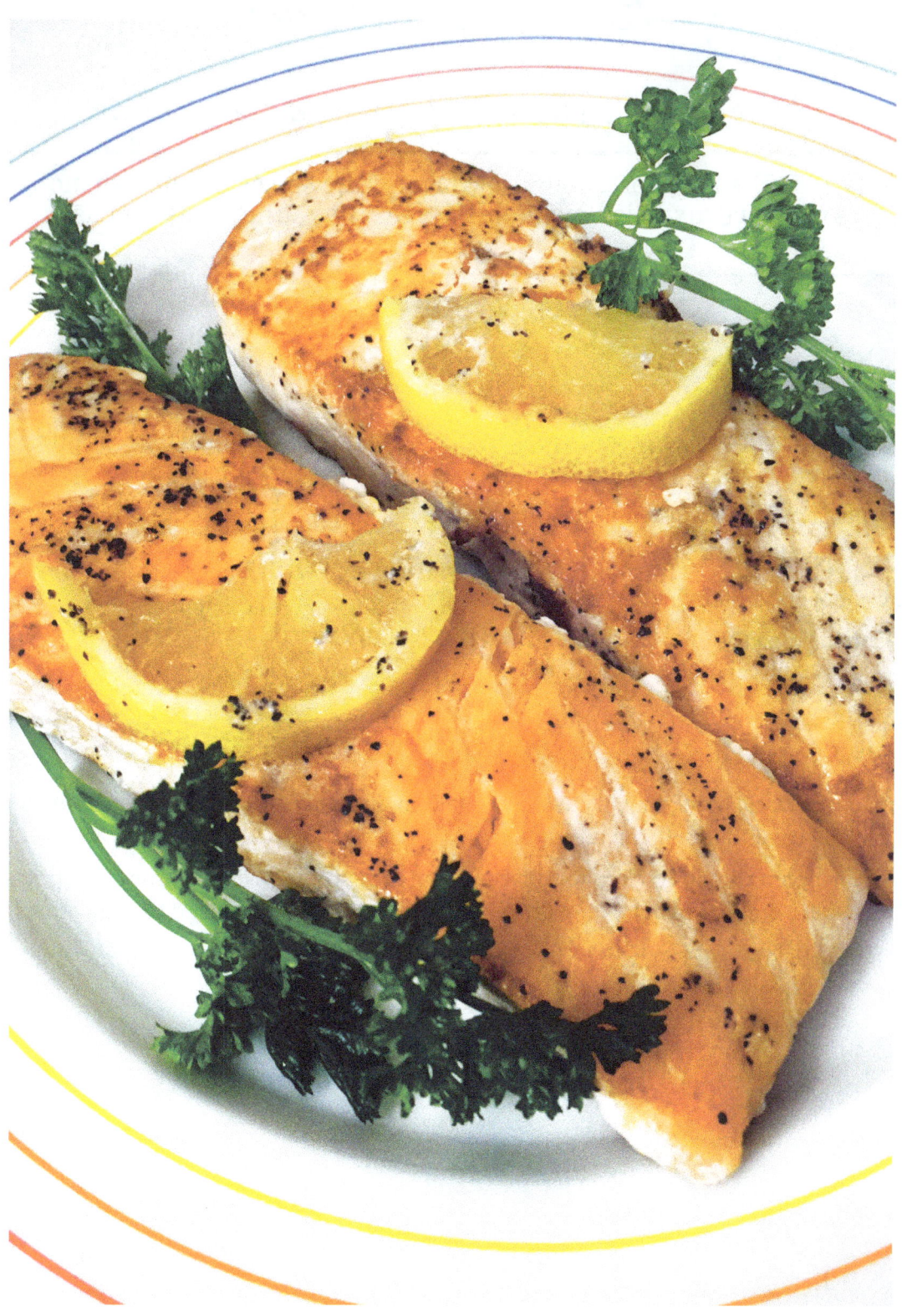

Broiled Tilapia

with Zesty Mandarin Orange Relish

Give this white fish a colorful burst of flavor! The spices on the fish along with the flavors of the citrus relish make this a treat for your eyes as well as your taste buds.

MAKES 4 SERVINGS

INGREDIENTS

- 1 ¼ cups mandarin oranges, canned in natural juice
- 1 ½ tablespoon white wine vinegar
- ¼ cup chopped onion
- ¼ cup chopped tomato
- 1 teaspoon lime juice
- 2 teaspoons chopped fresh cilantro
- 4 (4-ounce) tilapia fillets
- ½ teaspoon ground cumin
- 1 teaspoon paprika
- ⅛ teaspoon black pepper

INSTRUCTIONS

1. Combine mandarin oranges, white wine vinegar, onion, tomato, lime juice, and cilantro in a small bowl. Set aside for 45 minutes.
2. Coat broiler pan with nonstick spray. Place fish on rack and sprinkle with cumin, paprika, and black pepper. Broil for about 8 minutes or until fish begins to flake when tested with a fork.
3. Serve relish over warm fish.

Fish

Lemon Pepper Halibut
with Linguine

The linguine and vegetables provide you with a hearty meal that goes great with the natural buttery consistency of the grilled halibut. The mixture of flavors, textures, and nutrients will leave you completely satisfied!

MAKES 4 SERVINGS

INGREDIENTS

- 4-ounces uncooked whole wheat linguini
- 4 (4-ounce) halibut fillets
- ½ cup plain nonfat yogurt
- ¼ cup light mayonnaise
- 1 small onion, chopped
- ½ teaspoon chopped dill
- ½ teaspoon lemon juice
- ½ teaspoon black pepper
- 1 cup halved snow peas
- 1 small red bell pepper, chopped

INSTRUCTIONS

1. Cook linguine according to package directions. Set aside.
2. Wrap each halibut fillet in aluminum foil and grill until cooked through.
3. While halibut is cooking, mix together yogurt, mayonnaise, onion, dill, lemon juice, and black pepper.
4. Combine linguine, yogurt mixture, snow peas, and red pepper. Toss gently.
5. Place linguini onto plate and top with halibut fillet.

Broiled Fish Fillets

with Mustard

The broiled fish fillets in this recipe are fresh and flakey and go great with brown rice and steamed veggies. Put your leftovers to use by making a fish sandwich with tartar sauce and sliced tomato for lunch the next day!

MAKES 4 SERVINGS

INGREDIENTS

- 4 (5-ounce) thin flounder fillets (approximately 1 ¼ pounds)
- 2 tablespoons Dijon mustard
- ¼ teaspoon black pepper
- 1 lemon, cut into wedges
- 2 tablespoons chopped fresh parsley, for garnish

INSTRUCTIONS

1. Preheat oven to broil. Prepare a baking sheet with nonstick spray.
2. Arrange fish fillets on baking sheet.
3. Spread Dijon mustard over fish fillets. Sprinkle with black pepper.
4. Place in broiler 3 inches from heat and broil 2-3 minutes until golden; do not overcook.
5. Serve with lemon wedges. Garnish with chopped parsley.

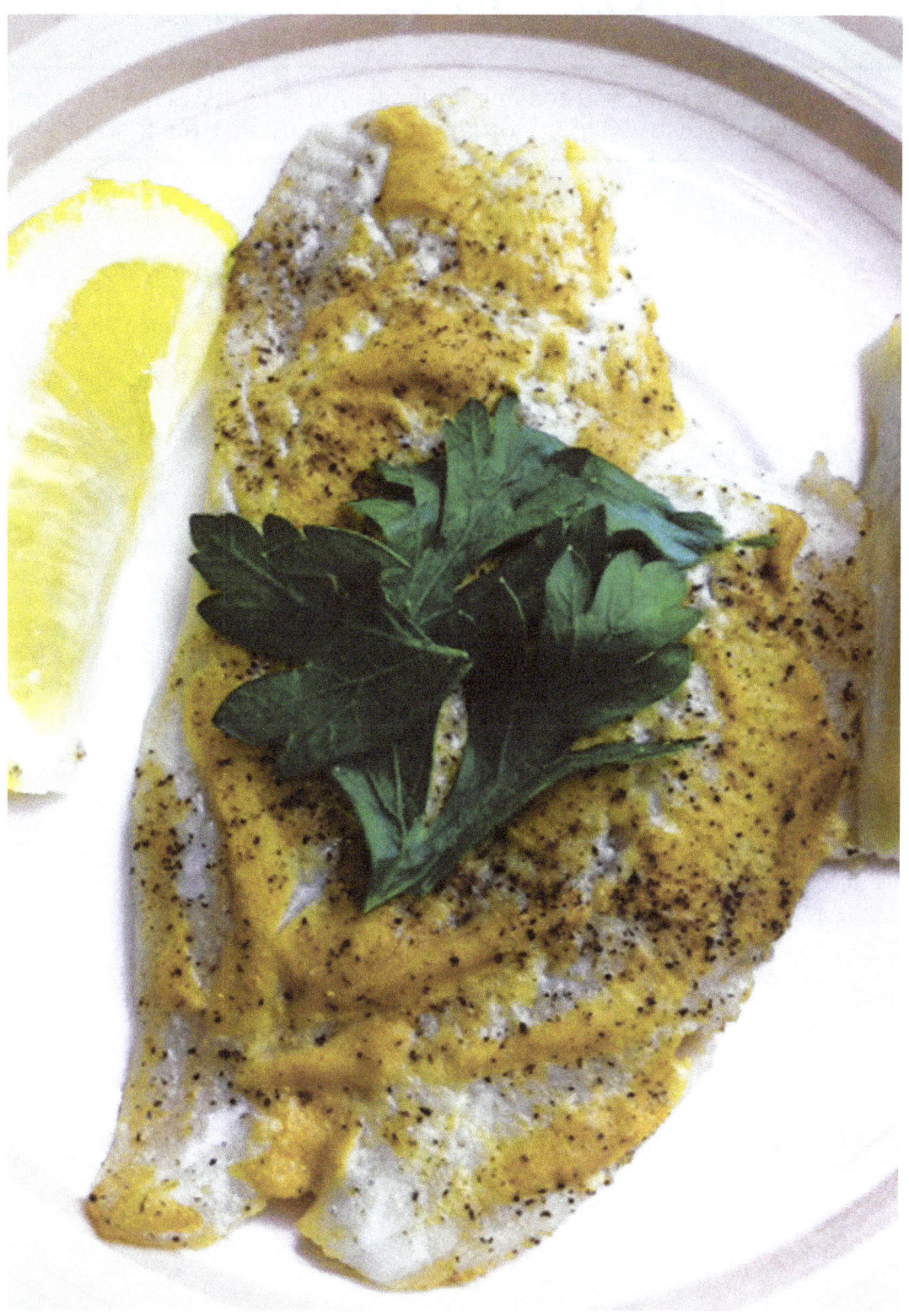

Orange-Glazed Salmon

This zesty salmon will have you tossing your take-out menus! These flavors come together to create a fresh Asian-style salmon dish that is better than ordering in.

MAKES 4 SERVINGS

INGREDIENTS

- ½ cup orange juice
- 1 tablespoon grated fresh ginger
- 2 teaspoons sesame oil
- 2 tablespoons low sodium soy sauce
- 1 pound center cut salmon fillets, cut into 4 fillets
- 1 tablespoon corn starch
- 2 tablespoons water

INSTRUCTIONS

1. Prepare a broiler pan with foil and nonstick spray.
2. In a medium bowl, combine orange juice, ginger, sesame oil, and soy sauce. Reserve ¼ cup to use for glaze.
3. Add salmon to the bowl. Cover and refrigerate 30 minutes.
4. Place salmon fillets in prepared broiler pan and broil or grill 15-20 minutes or until opaque in the center.
5. In a small saucepan, mix corn starch with water over low heat. Add reserved marinade and cook 1 minute until thickened.
6. Drizzle glaze over fillets.

Fish

Open-Faced Tuna Melt

What a delicious way to enjoy tuna…with cheese! Cheddar cheese melted over tuna with crunchy sweet pickles and red onion between whole wheat bread makes this sandwich even tastier. This dish pairs well with a green salad and a tall glass of unsweetened iced tea.

MAKES 4 SERVINGS

INGREDIENTS

- 2 (6-ounce) cans tuna, in water, drained
- ½ cup shredded carrots
- ¼ cup minced red onion
- ¼ cup light mayonnaise
- 1 sweet pickle, diced
- 1 teaspoon Dijon mustard
- ¼ teaspoon black pepper
- 4 slices whole wheat bread
- 4-ounces low fat shredded cheddar cheese

INSTRUCTIONS

1. Preheat broiler.
2. In a medium bowl, combine tuna, carrots, red onion, mayonnaise, pickles, mustard, and black pepper. Mix well.
3. Arrange bread slices on a baking sheet. Divide tuna mixture evenly on bread and top with shredded cheese.
4. Broil for 3-5 minutes, until cheese is bubbly.

Vegetable & Fish Stir-Fry

This stir-fry is fresh and satisfying with crunchy vegetables and tender fish. Flavorful yet versatile, pair this stir-fry with whole wheat noodles or brown rice for a complete meal.

MAKES 6 SERVINGS

INGREDIENTS

- 1 ½ tablespoons olive oil, divided
- 1 pound orange roughy (or sea bass), skin removed and cut into 1 ½-inch pieces
- 1 clove garlic, minced
- 1 shallot, minced
- 1 cup chopped red bell pepper
- 1 cup sliced celery
- 2 cups fresh snow peas, trimmed
- 1 cup sliced water chestnuts
- ½ cup fresh orange juice
- 2 teaspoons corn starch
- 1 teaspoon sesame oil
- 1 teaspoon rice vinegar
- 1 teaspoon low sodium soy sauce
- Chopped scallions, for garnish

INSTRUCTIONS

1. Heat 1 tablespoon olive oil in a wok or heavy skillet over medium-high heat.
2. Add fish and stir-fry gently until opaque, about 2-3 minutes. Remove fish from skillet and set aside.
3. Add remaining ½ tablespoon oil; stir-fry garlic and shallot for about 1 minute.
4. Add red pepper, celery, snow peas, and water chestnuts. Cover pan and steam 2 minutes.
5. Meanwhile, in a small dish, combine orange juice, corn starch, sesame oil, rice vinegar, and soy sauce. Add mixture to pan and cook until sauce thickens, about 1 minute.
6. Add fish back to pan and cook 1 minute. Garnish with chopped scallions before serving.

Tuna Boats

This is a fun recipe that you will enjoy making with your kids. The red pepper "boat" holds the tuna. Add carrots and celery for a healthy and creative eye catching lunch!

MAKES 4 SERVINGS

INGREDIENTS

- 1 (7-ounce) can tuna, in water, drained
- 1 tablespoon light mayonnaise
- 1 tablespoon low fat milk
- 2 small red bell peppers, cut in half

INSTRUCTIONS

1. In a bowl, mix tuna with mayonnaise and milk.
2. Remove seeds and membrane of peppers; fill with tuna mixture.

*Add shredded carrots or chopped celery to tuna mixture for added flavor. Carrots, thinly sliced lengthwise, cut into triangles make fun sails.

Intuitive Eating Wisdom

Intuitive Eating Principle 6: Discover the Satisfaction Factor

Food is meant to be enjoyed. When your mind is preoccupied with dieting, you lose sight of one of the simplest pleasures in life: the experience of eating. When you're eating food you enjoy without fear, you allow yourself to feel happy and satisfied. Rediscover the pleasure in all foods through intuitive eating.

Dairy & Pasta Entrees

IN THIS CHAPTER

207 | Spinach Parmesan Lasagna

208 | Shakshuka

210 | Vegetable Strata

211 | Broccoli Quiche

212 | Pita Pizza

214 | Cheesy Artichoke & Tomato Frittata

215 | Tomato Zucchini Parmesan

216 | Eggplant Casserole

218 | Fettuccini with Vegetables

Spinach Parmesan Lasagna

This unique twist on an Italian classic packs in extra flavor and nutrients! Rolled lasagna noodles are filled with spinach, mushrooms, cottage cheese, and seasonings topped with whole fresh crushed tomatoes and parmesan cheese. Accompany these delicious lasagna roll-ups with a side salad to complete the meal!

MAKES 4 SERVINGS

INGREDIENTS

- 2 (10-ounce) bags spinach leaves
- ¼ pound sliced fresh mushrooms
- 1 cup low fat cottage cheese
- ¼ teaspoon ground nutmeg
- ⅛ teaspoon black pepper
- 1 clove garlic, minced
- ½ cup chopped onion
- 8 cooked lasagna noodles
- 2 cups pureed whole tomatoes
- ½ teaspoon dried basil
- ½ teaspoon dried oregano
- 2 tablespoons grated Parmesan cheese

INSTRUCTIONS

1. Preheat oven to 350°F. Prepare a shallow baking dish with nonstick spray and set aside.
2. Steam the spinach until limp, then chop.
3. In a bowl, combine chopped spinach with mushrooms, cottage cheese, nutmeg, black pepper, garlic, and onion.
4. Line each lasagna noddle with 2 tablespoons of spinach mixture.
5. Roll up lasagna noodles and place in baking dish, standing on end.
6. Combine the pureed tomatoes, basil, and oregano in a bowl and pour over the noodles.
7. Sprinkle lightly with Parmesan cheese and bake for 40 minutes.

Shakshuka

Shakshuka is a staple dish in Middle Eastern cuisine that is comprised of eggs poached in a flavorful tomato sauce full of onions, peppers, and a variety of spices. The traditional ingredients in this recipe offer a ton of flavor and health benefits that can be eaten for any meal!

MAKES 6 SERVINGS

INGREDIENTS

- 1 clove garlic, chopped
- 1 medium onion, diced
- ½ medium red bell pepper, chopped
- ½ medium yellow bell pepper, chopped
- 1 tablespoon olive oil
- 3 large tomatoes, chopped
- 1 (14-ounce) can diced tomatoes
- 1 teaspoon chopped fresh basil
- ½ teaspoon paprika
- ½ teaspoon oregano
- ½ teaspoon ground cumin
- ½ teaspoon turmeric
- ¼ teaspoon black pepper
- 6 whole eggs
- Fresh basil, for garnish

INSTRUCTIONS

1. Sauté garlic, onion, and red and yellow peppers in olive oil for 5 minutes.
2. Add fresh tomatoes and sauté until tender, about 7 minutes.
3. Add canned tomatoes. Continue to sauté another 10 minutes, until sauce begins to thicken slightly.
4. Add basil, paprika, oregano, cumin, turmeric, and black pepper.
5. Place eggs into pan one-by-one. Cover and cook about 20-25 minutes until eggs are set.
6. Garnish with fresh basil.

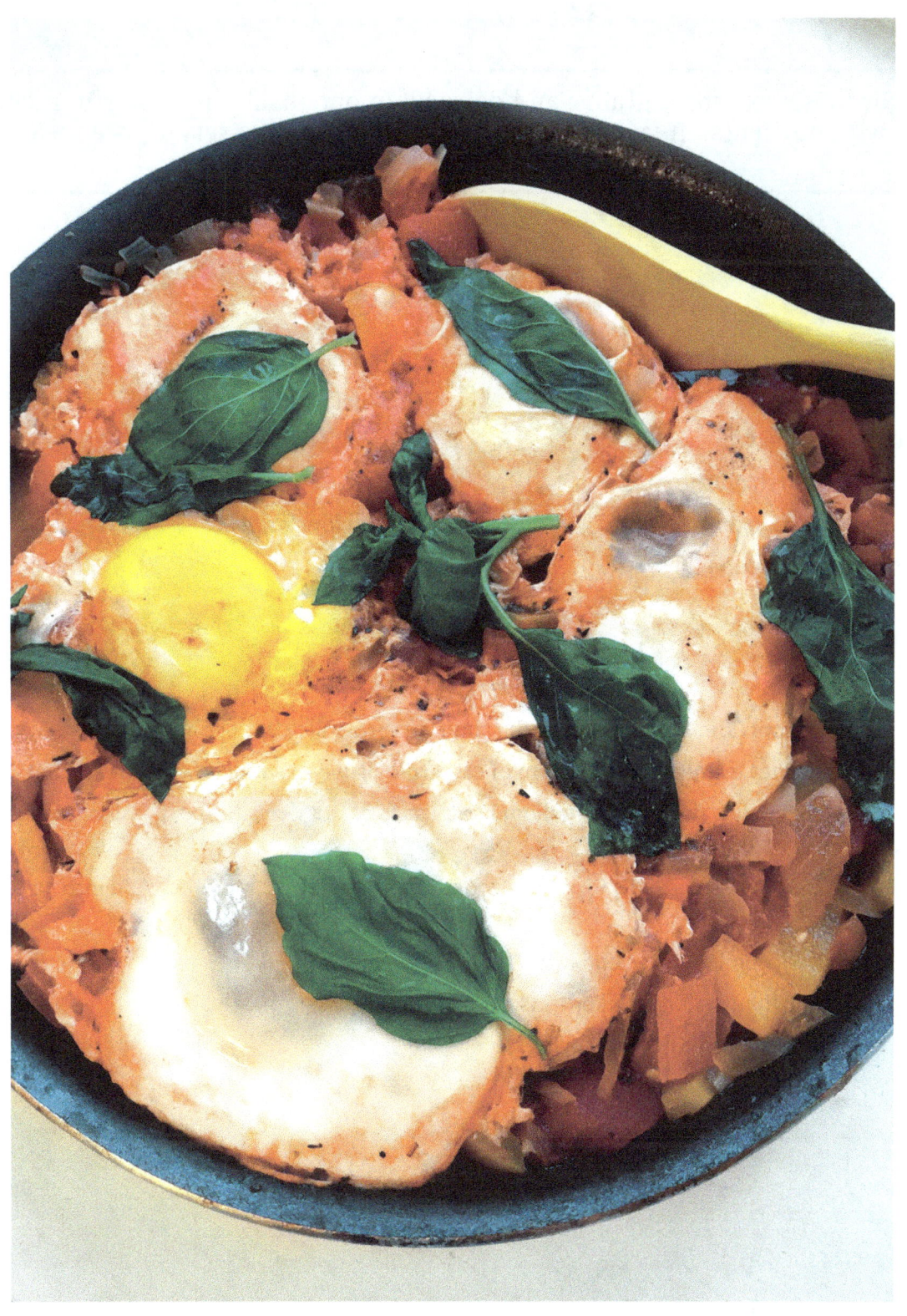

Vegetable Strata

Get your veggies, whole grains, and dairy all in one dish! This colorful recipe is filled with nutrients. It is creamy and smooth and can be served as a meal or an appetizer.

MAKES 6 SERVINGS

INGREDIENTS

- 2 slices whole wheat bread, cubed
- ¼ cup shredded low fat Swiss cheese
- ½ cup sliced carrots
- ½ cup sliced fresh mushrooms
- ¼ cup chopped onion
- 1 clove garlic, crushed
- 1 teaspoon olive oil
- ½ cup chopped tomato
- ½ cup snow peas
- 4 eggs
- ¾ cup low fat milk

INSTRUCTIONS

1. Preheat oven to 375°F. Prepare a 10-inch round casserole dish with nonstick spray.
2. Place bread cubes evenly on the bottom of casserole dish and sprinkle with cheese; set aside.
3. In a medium nonstick skillet over medium heat, sauté carrots, mushrooms, onion, and garlic in olive oil until tender.
4. Stir in chopped tomatoes and snow peas; cook for additional 1-2 minutes. Add into casserole dish.
5. In a small bowl, combine eggs and milk. Pour over vegetable mixture.
6. Bake for 45-50 minutes or until knife inserted in center comes out clean.
7. Let stand for 10 minutes before serving.

Broccoli Quiche

This recipe works as an easy side dish for dinner that will compliment any main course. A combination of simple ingredients like broccoli, cottage cheese, and mushrooms makes this quiche soft, tender, and nutritious.

MAKES 8 SERVINGS

INGREDIENTS

- 1 ½ heads of broccoli
- 8-ounces canned mushrooms
- 4-ounces shredded low fat mozzarella cheese
- 4-ounces low fat cottage cheese
- 1 whole egg
- 2 egg whites

INSTRUCTIONS

1. Preheat oven to 350°F.
2. Steam and mash broccoli.
3. In a medium bowl, combine broccoli, mushrooms, mozzarella cheese, cottage cheese, egg, and egg whites, mixing well.
4. Pour mixture into quiche dish and bake for 45 minutes.

Pita Pizza

Ditch take-out this weekend and make your own mini pizzas at home. Incorporating frozen spinach into this recipe makes it easy to get in a serving of greens. Do pizza your way and get your whole family involved in making dinner – your kids will love it!

MAKES 6 SERVINGS

INGREDIENTS

- 1 (10-ounce) box frozen chopped spinach, thawed, and strained
- 4-ounces light cream cheese
- 1 cup low fat ricotta cheese
- 2 tablespoons grated Parmesan cheese
- ¼ teaspoon garlic powder
- 6 (6-inch) whole wheat pita breads
- 6 plum tomatoes, each sliced into 6 slices

INSTRUCTIONS

1. Preheat broiler.
2. In a medium bowl, combine spinach, cream cheese, ricotta cheese, Parmesan cheese, and garlic powder; mix well.
3. Spread the mixture over pitas and top with tomato slices, dividing equally.
4. Place on a large rimmed baking sheet and broil for 4-5 minutes or until heated through. Serve immediately.

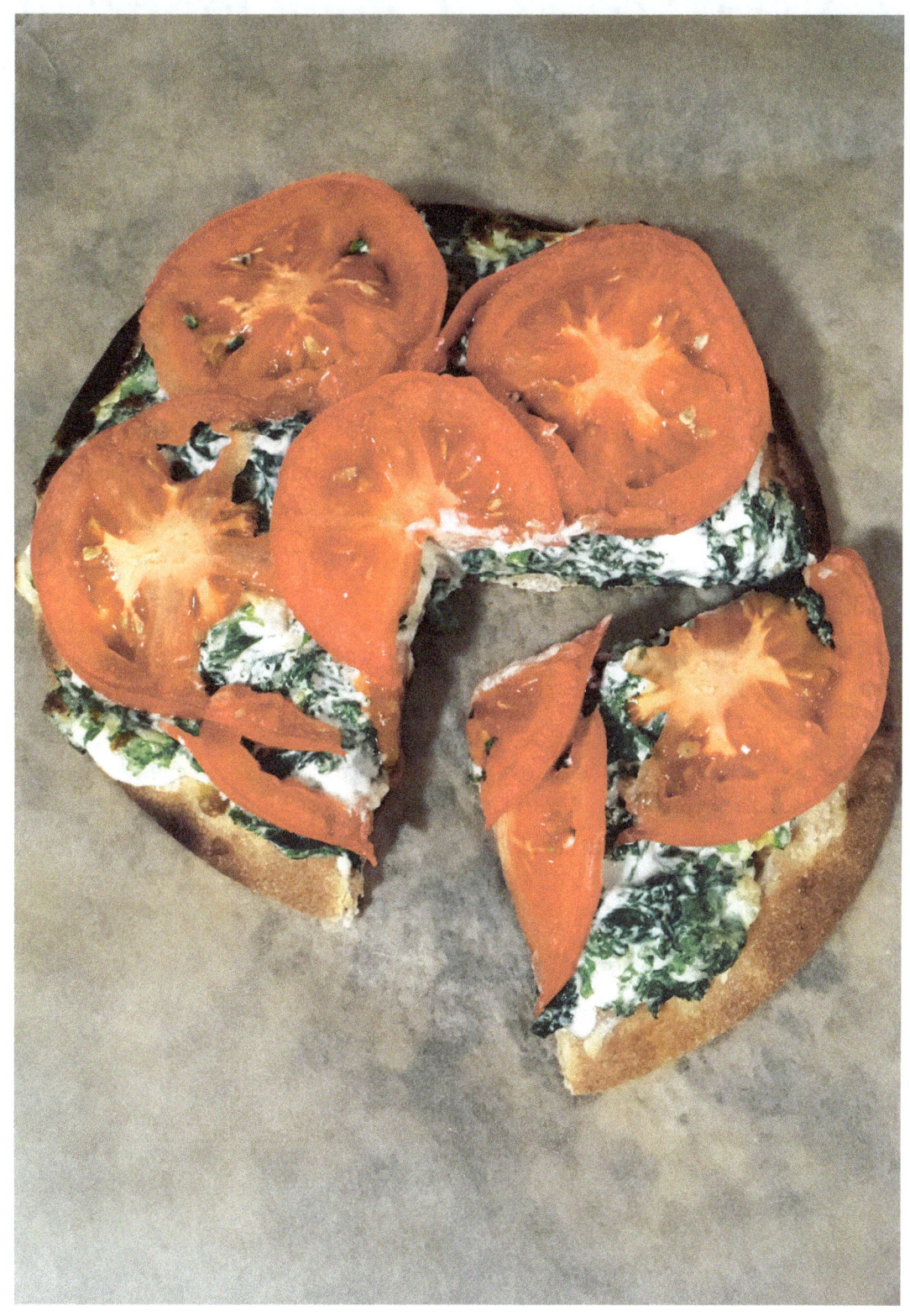

Cheesy Artichoke & Tomato Frittata

Fresh vegetables, fluffy eggs, and creamy cheese come together for an ultimate Sunday brunch frittata! Compliment with whole wheat toast and a fruit salad to make for a wholesome weekend meal.

MAKES 8 SERVINGS

INGREDIENTS

- 3 whole eggs
- 3 egg whites
- 3 tablespoons low fat milk
- ½ cup broccoli florets
- 2 tablespoons grated Parmesan cheese
- 2-ounces shredded low fat cheddar cheese
- ¼ teaspoon salt
- ¼ teaspoon black pepper
- 1 (14-ounce) can artichoke hearts, drained, coarsely chopped
- 1 tablespoon chopped fresh parsley
- 1 tablespoon chopped fresh basil
- 2 medium tomatoes, chopped

INSTRUCTIONS

1. In a medium bowl, combine eggs, eggs whites, milk, broccoli, Parmesan cheese, cheddar cheese, salt, and black pepper. Beat with wire whisk until well blended.
2. Spray medium nonstick ovenproof skillet with nonstick spray and place over medium-low heat.
3. Arrange artichokes in skillet, carefully pour egg mixture over artichokes, and sprinkle with parsley.
4. Cover and cook for 10-15 minutes or until eggs are set, but still moist on top.
5. Arrange chopped basil and tomatoes over egg mixture and serve!

Tomato Zucchini Parmesan

The zucchini and tomatoes add a smooth and tender texture plus extra vitamins to this dish. This family-friendly recipe is perfect for Sunday night dinner or an easy weeknight fix.

MAKES 6 SERVINGS

INGREDIENTS

- 2 cups thinly sliced green zucchini
- 2 cups thinly sliced yellow zucchini
- ¾ cup chopped onion
- 1 teaspoon olive oil
- ¼ cup chopped fresh parsley
- ½ teaspoon salt
- ¼ teaspoon garlic powder
- ½ teaspoon black pepper
- ¼ teaspoon dried basil
- ⅛ teaspoon oregano
- 1 cup halved cherry tomatoes
- 1 whole egg
- 2 egg whites
- 8-ounces shredded low fat mozzarella cheese
- 6-ounces pasta sauce

INSTRUCTIONS

1. Preheat oven to 375°F. Prepare a 12 x 8-inch baking dish with nonstick spray and set aside.
2. Spray a skillet with nonstick spray. Sauté zucchini and onions in olive oil until tender. Stir in parsley, salt, garlic powder, black pepper, dried basil, oregano, and tomatoes.
3. Beat egg and egg whites in a medium bowl. Add cheese, zucchini-onion mixture, and pasta sauce. Mix well.
4. Pour mixture into prepared baking dish and bake for 18-20 minutes or until set.
5. Let cool for 10 minutes before serving.

Eggplant Casserole

When it comes to eating vegetables, variety is always key! This recipe is no exception with ingredients like eggplant, tomatoes, zucchini, onion, peppers, and potatoes. The fresh flavors of the various vegetables in this recipe blend together in this light and tasty casserole.

MAKES 6 SERVINGS

INGREDIENTS

- 1 medium eggplant (approximately 1 ¼ pounds), sliced in ¼-inch rounds
- ½ teaspoon black pepper
- 2 tablespoons olive oil
- 3 cloves garlic, finely chopped
- ½ cup bread crumbs
- ¼ cup grated Parmesan cheese
- 8-ounces shredded low fat mozzarella cheese
- 3 medium potatoes, peeled, sliced in ¼-inch rounds
- 1 green bell pepper, sliced into ½-inch strips
- 1 red bell pepper, sliced into ½-inch strips
- 1 medium yellow onion, sliced into ½-inch rings
- 1 medium zucchini, sliced
- 1 (28-ounce) can whole peeled tomatoes in juice

INSTRUCTIONS

1. Preheat oven to 400°F. Prepare a large baking dish with nonstick spray.
2. Arrange eggplant slices on baking dish; sprinkle with black pepper, olive oil, ¼ of the garlic, 2 tablespoons bread crumbs, 1 tablespoon Parmesan cheese, and ¼ of the mozzarella cheese.
3. Arrange potato slices over eggplant slices. Again, sprinkle ¼ of the garlic, 2 tablespoons bread crumbs, 1 tablespoon parmesan cheese, and ¼ of the mozzarella cheese.
4. Place green peppers, red peppers, yellow onion and zucchini on top of potato slices. Top with peeled tomatoes and the rest of the garlic, bread crumbs, parmesan cheese and mozzarella cheese.
5. Bake for 45 minutes to an hour.

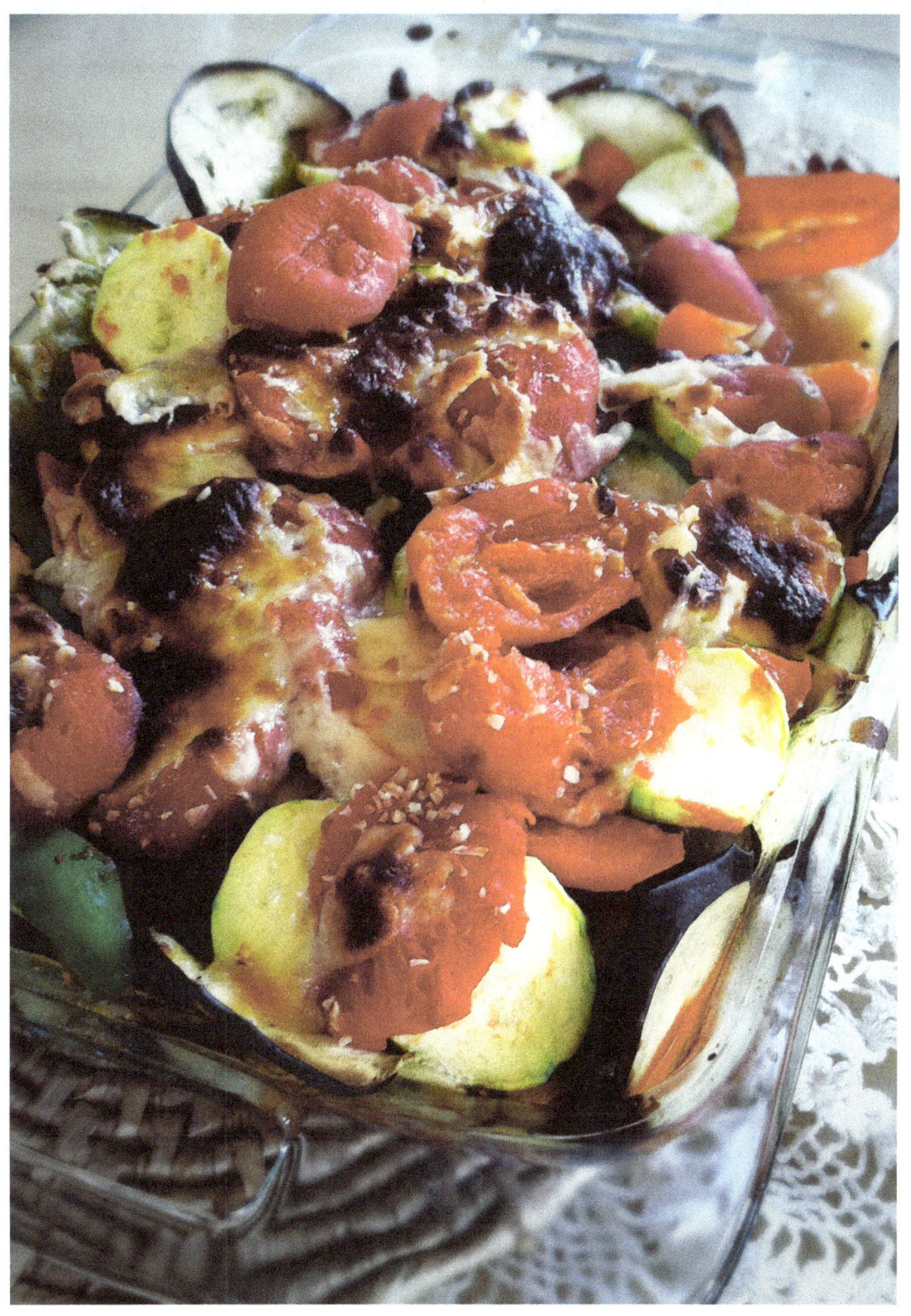

Fettuccini with Vegetables

Tender vegetables are tossed in creamy whole wheat fettuccini to create the perfect meal to keep you feeling satisfied. Pair with spinach salad topped with Feta cheese for a complete and balanced meal.

MAKES 5 SERVINGS

INGREDIENTS

- 2 cloves garlic
- 1 teaspoon olive oil
- 1 cup broccoli florets
- 1 cup sliced carrots
- 1 cup sliced zucchini
- ½ pound uncooked whole wheat fettuccine
- 1 teaspoon butter
- 2 teaspoons whole wheat flour
- ½ cup low sodium vegetable broth
- 2 tablespoons plain soy milk

INSTRUCTIONS

1. In a large saucepan prepared with nonstick spray, sauté garlic in olive oil until garlic browns. Add broccoli, carrots, and zucchini to saucepan and sauté until vegetables are tender. Set aside.
2. Cook fettuccine according to package directions and set aside.
3. In a small saucepan, melt butter over low heat. Add whole wheat flour and stir until a paste begins to form.
4. Add vegetable broth and stir thoroughly. Slowly stir in soy milk. Continue cooking on medium heat until liquid thickens, stirring constantly.
5. Mix vegetables with cooked fettuccine and toss with sauce.

Intuitive Eating Wisdom

Intuitive Eating Principle 7:
Cope with Your Emotions without Using Food

While it may act as a short-term distraction, food does not solve the underlying problems or feelings you may have. Recognizing emotional hunger versus physical hunger will allow you to learn how to meet your emotional needs without food.

Vegetarian

IN THIS CHAPTER

- 223 | Tofu-Stuffed Manicotti Shells
- 224 | Orzo-Stuffed Peppers
- 226 | Tempeh Fajitas
- 227 | Vegetable Cutlets
- 228 | Tofu Veggie Burgers
- 230 | Lentil-Stuffed Tomatoes
- 231 | Spicy Bean Burgers
- 232 | Tofu Crisp Over Noodles
- 234 | Mediterranean Veggie Burgers
- 235 | Tofu Chili

Vegetarian

Tofu-Stuffed Manicotti Shells

Try a new take on stuffed manicotti shells. In this recipe, tofu is perfectly combined with the ricotta, mozzarella, and Italian spices to add lean protein to this indulgent dish!

MAKES 12 SERVINGS

INGREDIENTS

- 1 (14-ounce) block light firm tofu, mashed
- 6-ounces shredded low fat mozzarella cheese
- 8-ounces low fat ricotta cheese
- ¼ cup chopped fresh parsley
- 1 tablespoon onion powder
- 1 teaspoon garlic powder
- ¼ teaspoon salt
- ½ teaspoon black pepper
- ½ teaspoon dried basil
- 1 (27-ounce) jar pasta sauce
- 12 jumbo cooked manicotti shells
- ¼ cup grated Parmesan cheese

INSTRUCTIONS

1. Preheat oven to 350°F. Prepare a 9 x 9-inch baking dish with nonstick spray and set aside.
2. Combine tofu, mozzarella cheese, ricotta cheese, parsley, onion powder, garlic powder, salt, black pepper, and basil in a medium bowl; set the mixture aside.
3. Spread 2 cups of pasta sauce in the bottom of prepare baking dish. Fill each shell with the tofu mixture. Arrange stuffed shells in the baking dish.
4. Spoon the remaining sauce over filled shells and sprinkle with Parmesan cheese.
5. Bake for 25-30 minutes, until lightly browned and bubbly.

Orzo-Stuffed Peppers

Orzo is a great substitute for rice or pasta that will add variety to your meals. Experiment with orzo in this stuffed pepper recipe that combines the fresh flavors of peppers, thyme, onions, and parsley.

MAKES 6 SERVINGS

INGREDIENTS

- 8-ounces uncooked orzo
- 2 teaspoons olive oil
- 2 cloves garlic, minced
- 1 medium onion, chopped
- 1 stalk celery, diced
- ½ teaspoon, thyme
- 1 tablespoon chopped fresh parsley
- ½ cup grated Parmesan cheese
- 2 cups low sodium vegetable broth
- 3-ounces shredded low fat mozzarella cheese
- 2 medium-large red bell peppers
- 2 medium-large green bell peppers
- 2 medium-large yellow bell peppers
- 3 teaspoons bread crumbs

INSTRUCTIONS

1. Preheat oven to 350°F.
2. Prepare orzo according to package directions and set aside.
3. Heat oil in medium saucepan; add garlic, onion, and celery. Cover and cook vegetables until soft. Remove from heat. Stir in orzo, thyme, parsley, Parmesan cheese, ½ cup of the vegetable broth, and ½ of the mozzarella cheese.
4. Cut tops off peppers and remove seeds. Cut a small piece off the bottoms so peppers will stand upright. Stand peppers in a baking dish. Spoon the orzo mixture into each pepper.
5. Sprinkle the top of each pepper with ½ teaspoon bread crumbs and the remaining ½ of the mozzarella cheese. Pour the remaining 1 ½ cups of broth around the peppers.
6. Bake for 45 minutes, or until tender and lightly browned on top. Serve immediately.

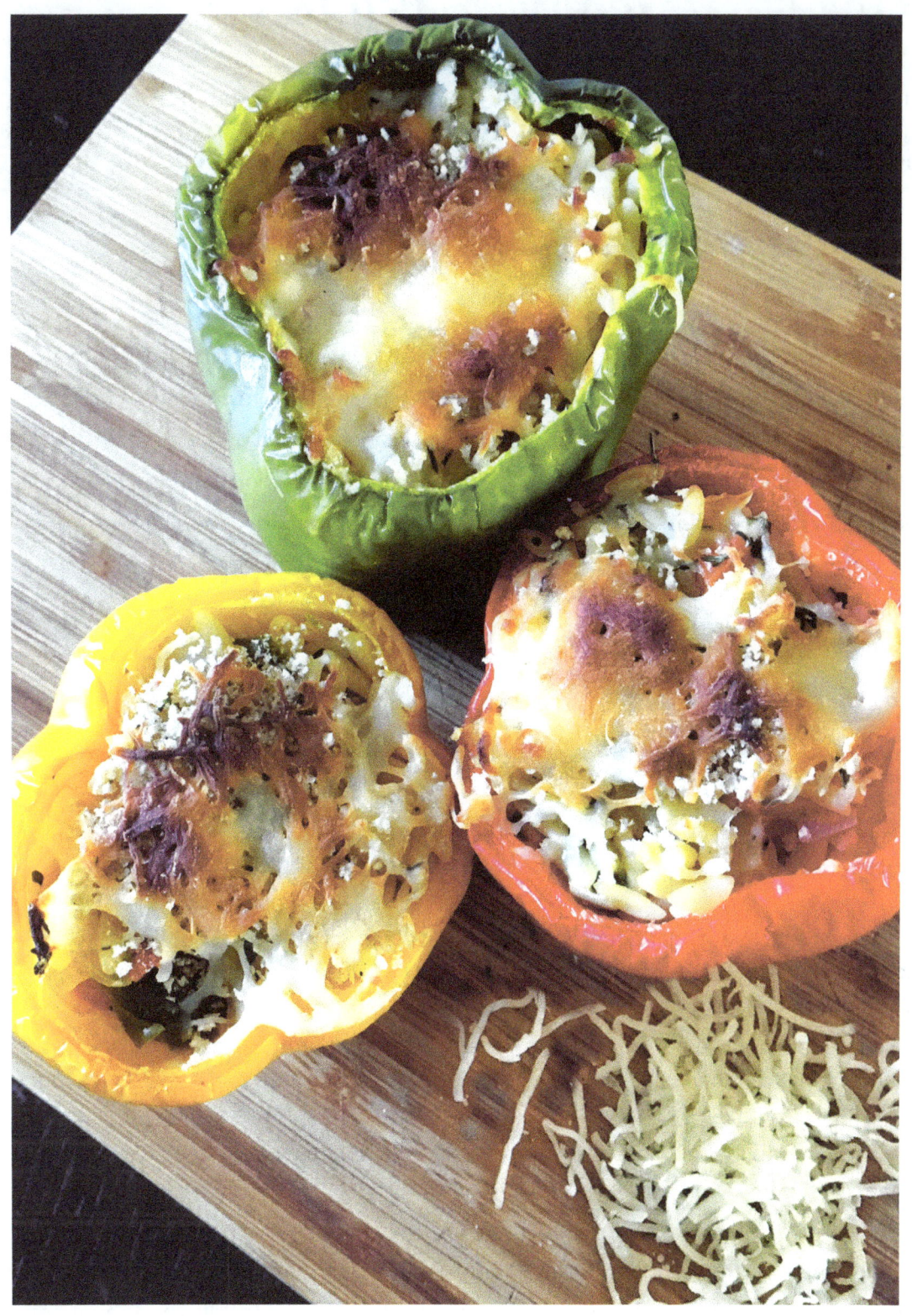

Tempeh Fajitas

Tempeh is a plant-based protein that is as versatile as meat. This recipe blends Indian and Mediterranean flavors with tomatoes, red peppers, and onions. Fajitas at home is a fun way family to get the family involved in preparing their meal.

MAKES 12 SERVINGS

MARINADE INGREDIENTS

- 1 teaspoon olive oil
- 1 medium onion, finely chopped
- 3 cloves garlic, minced
- 1 tablespoon chili powder
- 1 teaspoon ground cumin
- 1 cup water
- 3 tablespoons lime juice
- ¼ teaspoon salt
- ¼ teaspoon black pepper
- 1 teaspoon oregano
- ⅛ teaspoon cayenne pepper

FAJITA INGREDIENTS

- 16-ounces tempeh, sliced ¾-inch thick
- 1 teaspoon olive oil
- 1 large red bell pepper, cut into ¼-inch slices
- 1 small red onion, cut into ¼-inch slices
- 1 small tomato, chopped
- 12 whole wheat tortillas

INSTRUCTIONS

1. In a medium saucepan, heat 1 teaspoon olive oil over medium heat. Sauté onion until it becomes translucent. Add garlic and continue cooking until lightly browned. Add chili powder and cumin and stir well.
2. Stir in water and lime juice until mixture develops a pasty texture. Add salt, black pepper, oregano, and cayenne pepper and mix well. Transfer to a dish and set aside. Once marinade is cooled, place tempeh slices in the dish and put in refrigerator for 2 hours.
3. Spray a medium skillet with nonstick spray. Heat 1 teaspoon olive oil and sauté red pepper, red onion, and tomato until onion is translucent. Set aside.
4. In the same pan, cook marinated tempeh for 2-3 minutes on each side.
5. In a medium skillet, heat tortillas turning every 5-7 seconds, until tortilla is hot and pliable.
6. Divide tempeh slices and cooked vegetables evenly and place on tortillas and serve hot.

Vegetarian

Vegetable Cutlets

These filling and flavorful vegetable cutlets will change the way you think of a traditional "cutlet"! They are meat-free and loaded with nutritious vegetables like peas, carrots, and potatoes – a fun and creative way to get in your daily serving of veggies!

MAKES 8 SERVINGS

INGREDIENTS

- 1 (9-ounce) package frozen green peas
- 3 medium carrots, diced and peeled
- 1 medium onion, sliced
- 2 medium potatoes, cubed
- 1 cup water
- ½ pound fresh spinach leaves
- 1 whole egg
- 2 egg whites
- 1 cup bread crumbs

INSTRUCTIONS

1. Preheat oven to 350°F. Prepare a baking dish with nonstick spray and set aside.
2. Boil peas, carrots, onion and potatoes in 1 cup of water.
3. Add spinach, cover and simmer until vegetables are soft and water is absorbed, about 8 minutes.
4. Remove from heat. Let stand for about 5 minutes or until cool.
5. Beat egg and egg whites in a small bowl. Add eggs and bread crumbs to vegetable mixture; mix well.
6. Form vegetable cutlets in the palm of your hand and place in prepared dish.
7. Bake in preheated oven for 20 minutes. Flip the cutlets and bake for an additional 20 minutes.

Tofu Veggie Burgers

Your family will love these flavorful veggies burgers and they won't even miss the meat! Packed with great taste, each veggie burger contains one full serving of vegetables. Enjoy on a whole wheat bun or atop a green salad.

MAKES 16 SERVINGS

INGREDIENTS

- 1 (14-ounce) block light firm tofu
- 2 tablespoons olive oil, divided
- 1 medium onion, diced
- 1 large carrot, grated
- 12 fresh white mushrooms, finely chopped
- 2 cups uncooked quick cooking oats
- ½ teaspoon onion powder
- 1 teaspoon garlic powder
- 2 teaspoons turmeric
- 1 cup water
- 1 cup seasoned bread crumbs

INSTRUCTIONS

1. Drain and crumble tofu in a large mixing bowl and set aside.
2. Heat a large skillet over medium heat and add 1 tablespoon olive oil. Sauté onion, carrots, and mushrooms until onions become translucent.
3. Add the oats, onion powder, garlic powder and turmeric to the sauté mixture. Continue cooking until the oats are toasted, approximately 5-6 minutes.
4. Add water and stir to combine.
5. Remove skillet from heat and stir in breadcrumbs. Let the mixture cool, then add it to the crumbled tofu and mix well.
6. Shape the mixture into patties. In a skillet sprayed with nonstick spray, cook patties until browned on each side.

Note: You can bake the mixture in a loaf pan for a delicious Tofu "meatloaf".

Vegetarian

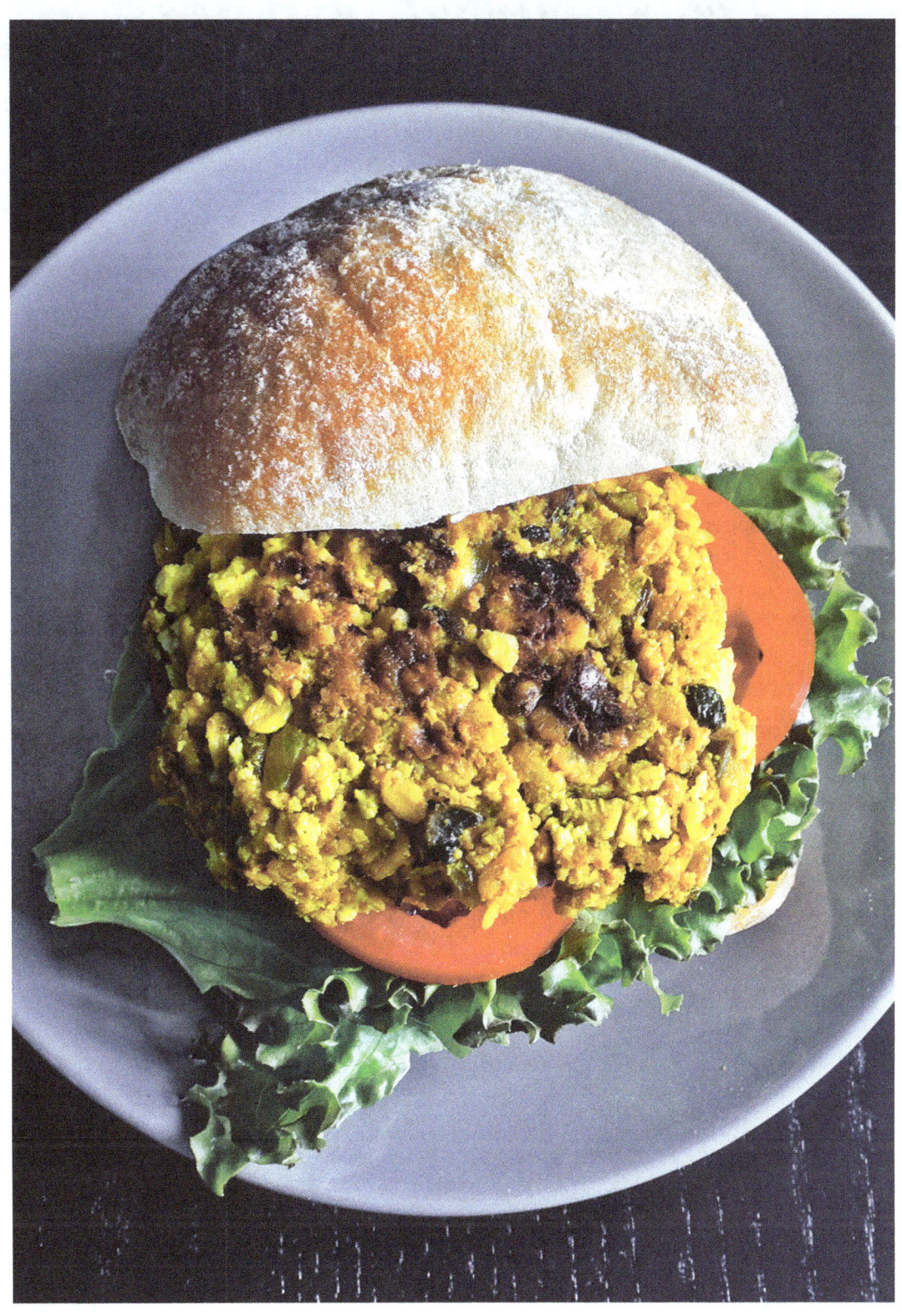

Lentil-Stuffed Tomatoes

In this recipe, lentils are mixed with fresh vegetables and stuffed in a juicy tomato for a perfectly light meal that will hit the spot! This dish might sound intimidating but it's easy to prepare and delicious.

MAKES 4 SERVINGS

INGREDIENTS

- 4 firm medium tomatoes
- ¼ cup chopped celery
- 2 cloves garlic, chopped
- ¼ cup chopped onion
- 2 tablespoons chopped green bell pepper
- ½ teaspoon curry powder
- ½ teaspoon salt
- 1 cup cooked brown lentils
- 1 tablespoon grated Parmesan cheese

INSTRUCTIONS

1. Preheat oven to 400°F.
2. Core the tomatoes; scoop the pulp and juice into a bowl and mash. Place the tomato shells, cut side down, on paper towels to drain.
3. In a medium saucepan, combine tomato pulp-juice mixture, celery, garlic, onion, green pepper, curry, and salt. Cook over medium heat, until vegetables are tender, approximately 5 minutes.
4. Add lentils and continue cooking until the mixture is thick and lentils are soft.
5. Place tomatoes on a baking sheet, cut side up. Divide the mixture evenly into the 4 tomato shells and sprinkle with Parmesan cheese.
6. Bake until heated through, about 10-15 minutes.

Vegetarian

Spicy Bean Burgers

These burgers have heat, but no meat! You'll love the added flavor brought on by the green peppers and onions. Enjoy this burger with baked sweet potato fries.

MAKES 4 SERVINGS

INGREDIENTS

- 1 (16-ounce) can dark red kidney beans, drained and rinsed
- 1 small red onion, finely chopped
- ½ green bell pepper, chopped
- 2 egg whites
- ¼ cup whole wheat bread crumbs
- 2 cloves garlic, minced
- ¼ cup finely chopped fresh parsley
- 1 teaspoon chili pepper
- 1 tablespoon olive oil
- ½ cup shredded low fat mozzarella cheese

INSTRUCTIONS

1. In a large bowl, mash beans with a potato masher until mostly crushed. Add red onion, green pepper, egg whites, bread crumbs, garlic, parsley, and chili pepper and mix well.
2. With wet hands, shape mixture into four ½-inch thick patties.
3. Spray a medium skillet with nonstick spray. Place over medium-high heat and add olive oil. Arrange patties in skillet and cook for 3-4 minutes on each side or until patties are heated through and slightly crusty.
4. Reduce to low heat; top each patty with cheese.
5. Cover skillet and cook for 1-2 minutes or until cheese begins to melt.

Tofu Crisp Over Noodles

This dish is perfect for those who are looking for a new way to enjoy tofu. The breadcrumbs add texture to the smooth consistency of the tofu. This crisp tofu can be an alternative protein to top noodles, salads, or mixed vegetables.

MAKES 4 SERVINGS

TOFU INGREDIENTS

- 1 (14-ounce) block extra-firm tofu
- ½ pound uncooked whole wheat noodles
- 2 tablespoons bread crumbs
- 1 teaspoon peanut oil

MARINADE INGREDIENTS

- ¼ cup rice vinegar
- ⅓ tablespoon low sodium soy sauce
- 1 tablespoon all-natural peanut butter
- 1 clove garlic, minced
- 2 tablespoons minced scallions
- 1 teaspoon chili paste or powder
- 1 tablespoon water
- 1 teaspoon sugar

INSTRUCTIONS

1. Cut block of tofu into quarters. Press out water using a towel.
2. Mix all marinade ingredients with a wire whisk or fork in a medium bowl. Place tofu in marinade for 15 minutes, then rotate and let marinate for another 15 minutes.
3. In the meantime, cook noodles according to package directions and set aside.
4. Dip the marinated tofu into bread crumbs to fully coat tofu. Reserve marinade. Spray medium skillet with nonstick spray and heat 1 teaspoon of peanut oil. Cook tofu until golden brown, approximately 1 ½ minutes on each side.
5. Heat remaining marinade mixture over the stove or in the microwave and pour over noodles. Place tofu crisp over noodles and serve.

Vegetarian

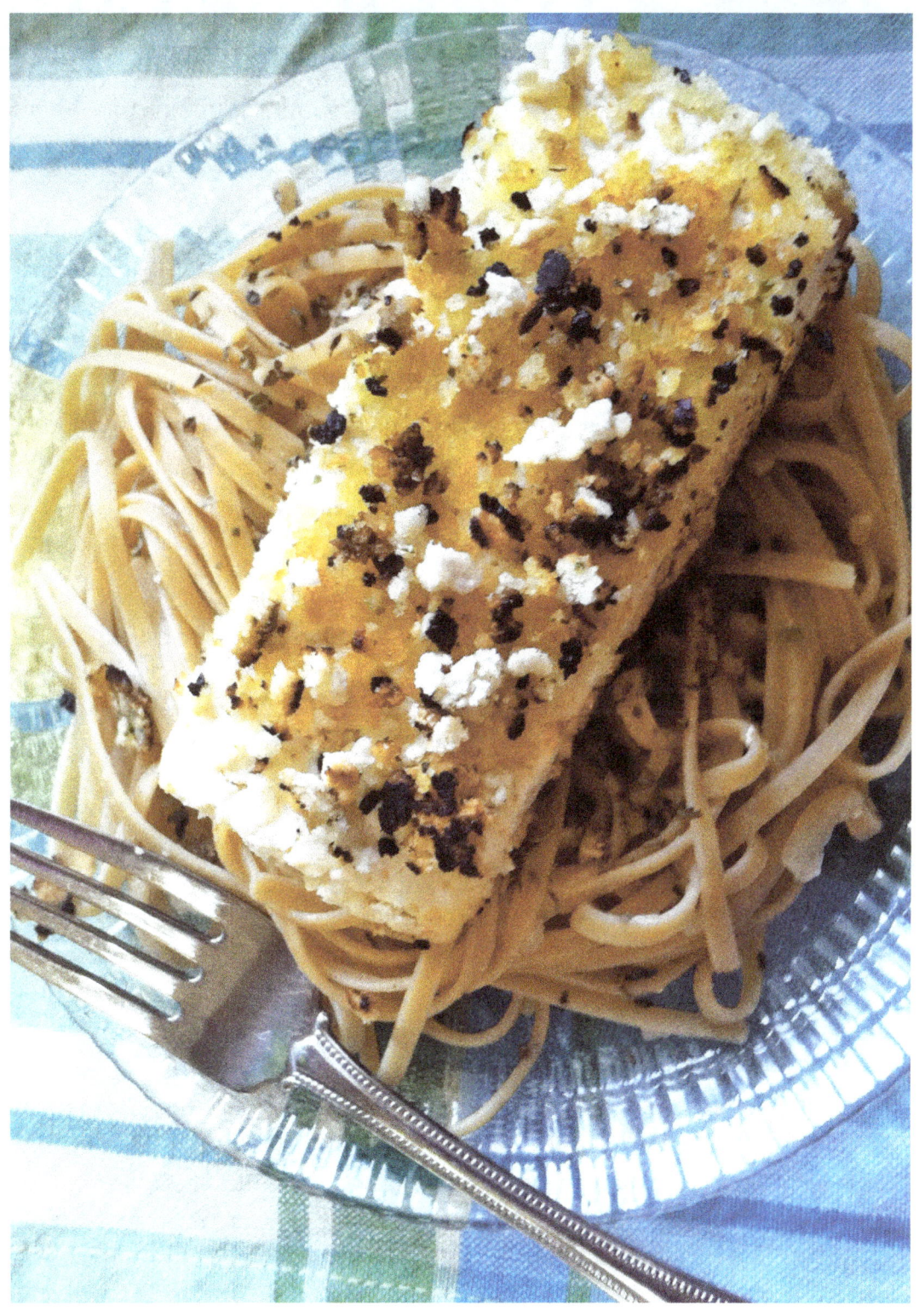

Mediterranean Veggie Burgers

Give burger night a vegetarian-friendly makeover! Not only are these burgers filled with nutrients that will satisfy your hunger, they are easy to make too. Vegetarians and meat-eaters alike will love these burgers.

MAKES 4 SERVINGS

INGREDIENTS

- ¼ cup plain nonfat Greek yogurt
- 2 tablespoons Dijon mustard
- 1 tablespoon chopped fresh parsley
- ½ teaspoon salt
- ½ teaspoon black pepper
- 1 (15-ounce) can chickpeas, drained and rinsed
- 1 cup cooked brown rice
- 1 teaspoon olive oil
- 1 medium green bell pepper, finely chopped
- 1 clove garlic, chopped
- 1 cup chopped scallions
- 3 tablespoons lemon juice
- 1 tablespoon olive oil
- 2 whole wheat pitas
- 1 medium tomato, sliced
- 4 Romaine lettuce leaves

INSTRUCTIONS

1. In a small mixing bowl, combine Greek yogurt, Dijon mustard, parsley, salt, and black pepper. Chill dressing in refrigerator for 1-2 hours.
2. In a medium bowl, mash chickpeas. Add brown rice and mix well. Set aside.
3. In a medium skillet, heat olive oil over medium heat. Sauté green pepper, garlic, and scallions until green pepper is soft.
4. Add sautéed mixture and lemon juice to chickpeas and brown rice and combine well. Shape into four ¾-inch thick patties.
5. Spray medium skillet with nonstick spray. Heat olive oil and cook patties for approximately 6 minutes each side or until browned and thoroughly heated.
6. Cut pitas in half. Tuck patties, tomato slices, lettuce leaves, and dressing into each pita.

Vegetarian

Tofu Chili

The sweet green pepper, rich tomato sauce, and starchy texture of the beans all combine well to make this dish unique. This tofu chili makes a great lunch; add a whole wheat roll as a dipper or accompany with a mixed green salad.

MAKES 8 SERVINGS

INGREDIENTS

- 2 cups firm tofu, cut into 1-inch cubes
- 1 clove garlic, minced
- 1 tablespoon chili powder
- 2 tablespoons Worcestershire sauce
- 1 medium onion, chopped
- 1 medium green bell pepper, chopped
- 2 stalks celery, chopped
- 1 medium tomato, chopped
- 1 (16-ounce) can tomato sauce
- 1 (15-ounce) can dark red kidney beans, drained and rinsed
- 1 (15-ounce) can white kidney beans, drained and rinsed
- ½ teaspoon dried basil
- ½ cup chopped scallions, for garnish

INSTRUCTIONS

1. In a medium bowl, combine tofu, garlic, chili powder and Worcestershire sauce; set aside.
2. Coat a large skillet with nonstick spray. Sauté onion, green pepper, and celery until onion becomes translucent.
3. Add tofu mixture; cook and stir gently for approximately 3 minutes.
4. Add tomato, tomato sauce, red and white kidney beans, and basil to skillet and mix well.
5. Cover and simmer over medium-low heat for 30 minutes.
6. Garnish with chopped scallions.

Intuitive Eating Wisdom

Intuitive Eating Principle 8: Respect Your Body

Love and appreciate your body and all that is does for you. This transformation will not come overnight but in the many small reminders that you'll have on your journey. Your body carries you through life and deserves care and respect. Freeing yourself of body worry will help release the food worry and stop the vicious cycle of dieting.

Breakfast

IN THIS CHAPTER

241 | Cheesy Egg Quesadillas

242 | Vegetable Tofu Scramble

244 | Veggie Egg Delight

245 | Banana Nut Pancakes

246 | Whole Wheat Chocolate Pancakes

248 | Fruit French Toast Casserole

Breakfast

Cheesy Egg Quesadillas

Treat yourself to a wholesome breakfast with these cheesy breakfast quesadillas. With vegetables, eggs, cheese, whole grains, spices, and herbs, this recipe starts your day with every food group.

MAKES 4 SERVINGS

INGREDIENTS

- 2 whole eggs
- 4 egg whites
- ½ cup diced red bell pepper
- ½ cup chopped cilantro
- ¼ cup shredded low fat Cheddar cheese
- ¼ teaspoon chili powder
- 4 soft whole wheat tortillas

INSTRUCTIONS

1. Coat a medium skillet with nonstick spray and heat over medium flame.
2. In a small bowl, whisk eggs and egg whites together.
3. Add red pepper, cilantro, Cheddar cheese, and chili powder to egg mixture.
4. Scramble egg mixture in skillet and cook until eggs are set.
5. Heat tortillas in skillet and add ½ cup scrambled eggs onto one side. Fold tortilla in half and heat until golden brown on each side.

Vegetable Tofu Scramble

This is a perfect high protein vegan breakfast that has sweet and crunchy bell peppers and a spicy salsa kick! Try it over lettuce or in a whole wheat wrap.

MAKES 3 SERVINGS

INGREDIENTS

- 1 (14-ounce) block light firm tofu
- ½ teaspoon olive oil
- 1 scallion, chopped
- 1 clove garlic, minced
- ½ cup diced red bell pepper
- ½ cup diced green bell pepper
- ⅓ cup salsa
- ½ teaspoon salt
- ½ teaspoon black pepper

INSTRUCTIONS

1. Drain tofu and wrap in a dish towel. Let stand for about 30 minutes then crumble into small pieces.
2. Heat olive oil in medium skillet. Sauté scallions and garlic until golden brown.
3. Add crumbled tofu, red pepper, green pepper, and salsa. Season with salt and black pepper. Mix well and heat through.

Breakfast

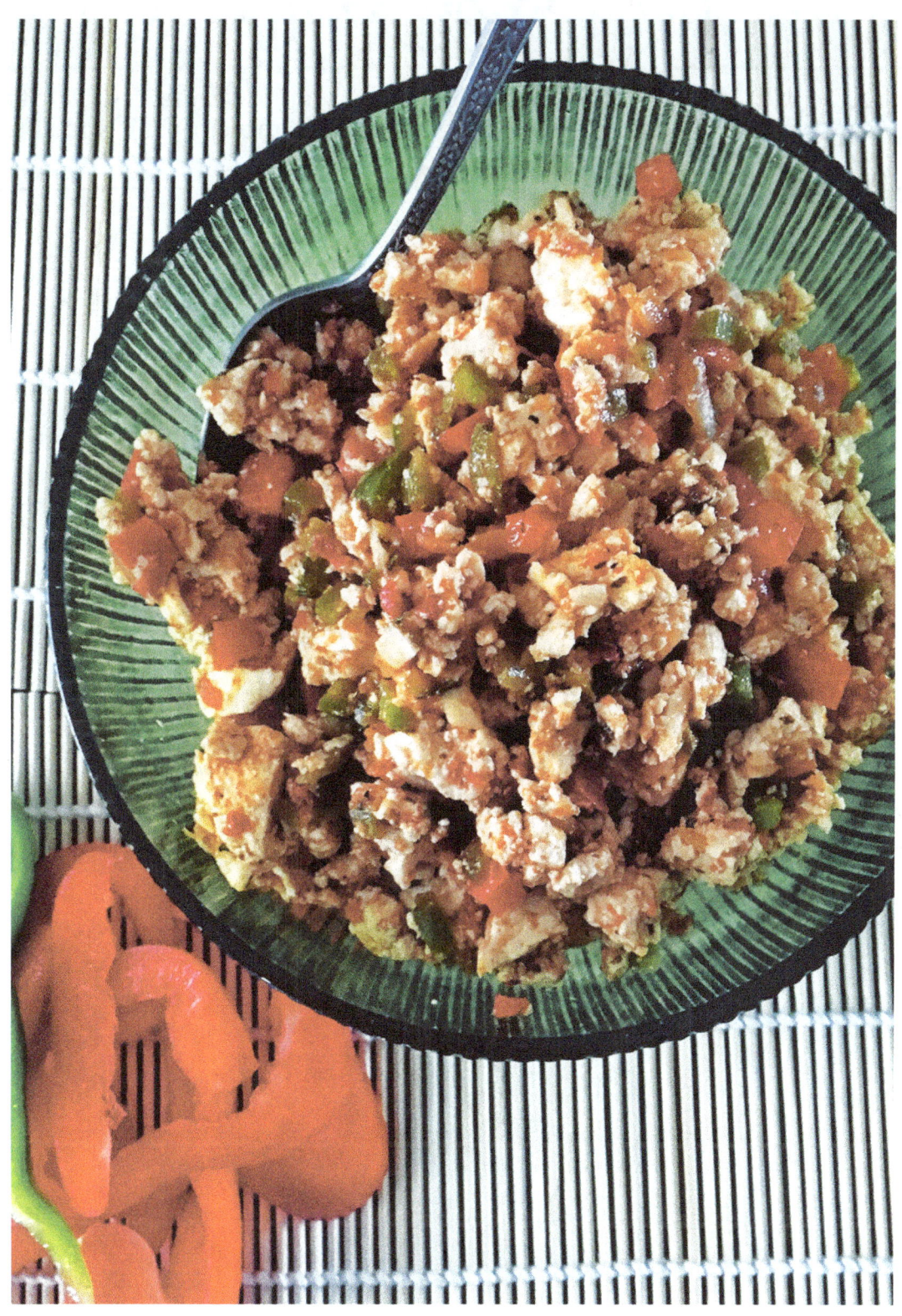

Veggie Egg Delight

This recipe will start your day with a colorful serving of vegetables. Pair these fluffy eggs and veggies with whole wheat toast and a piece of fruit and you will power through your morning.

MAKES 6 SERVINGS

INGREDIENTS

- 1 teaspoon olive oil
- 1 cup chopped onion
- 2 medium red bell peppers, chopped
- 1 cup chopped fresh mushrooms
- 1 cup broccoli florets
- 3 whole eggs
- 2 egg whites
- ⅓ cup low fat milk
- ¼ teaspoon salt
- ½ teaspoon black pepper
- 1-ounce shredded low fat mozzarella cheese

INSTRUCTIONS

1. Heat olive oil over medium heat in a nonstick pan.
2. Add onions and red pepper and cook for 10 minutes stirring constantly.
3. Add mushrooms and broccoli. Stir and cook for 5 more minutes.
4. Beat eggs and egg whites with milk and pour over vegetables. Season with salt and black pepper.
5. Cook for approximately 15 minutes or until bottom is nicely browned and omelet is puffy.
6. Sprinkle mozzarella cheese over the omelet and allow to melt.

Breakfast

Banana Nut Pancakes

These pancakes pack healthy goodness with the use of whole wheat flour and heart healthy olive oil and walnuts. The sweet flavor from the bananas and honey makes these pancakes anything but bland. A perfect recipe for a lazy weekend morning!

MAKES 10 SERVINGS

INGREDIENTS

- 1 ½ cups whole wheat flour
- 2 teaspoons baking powder
- ½ teaspoon salt
- 1 cup low fat milk
- 1 tablespoon olive oil
- 2 tablespoons honey
- 2 large bananas, mashed
- ½ cup chopped walnuts
- 2 egg whites

INSTRUCTIONS

1. In a medium bowl, combine whole wheat flour, baking powder, and salt.
2. Stir in milk, olive oil, honey, bananas, and walnuts.
3. Beat egg whites in a small bowl until frothy. Fold into pancake batter.
4. Heat a medium skillet with nonstick spray over medium heat.
5. Pour ¼ cup of pancake batter into skillet and cook until both sides are golden brown. Repeat with remaining batter.

Whole Wheat Chocolate Pancakes

Dessert meets breakfast in this hearty yet chocolate-rich pancake recipe! Enjoy these breakfast pancakes with berries and a glass of chilled milk.

MAKES 10 SERVINGS

INGREDIENTS

- 1 cup whole wheat flour
- ½ cup unsweetened cocoa powder
- 1 tablespoon sugar
- 2 teaspoons baking powder
- ¼ teaspoon salt
- 4 egg whites
- 1 ½ cups plain soy milk
- 2-ounces low fat dark chocolate squares, grated

INSTRUCTIONS

1. In a medium bowl, combine whole wheat flour, cocoa powder, sugar, baking powder, and salt.
2. In a separate bowl, lightly beat egg whites and add soy milk. Mix well.
3. Add wet ingredients to dry ingredients and mix until blended well. Add dark chocolate into mixture.
4. Heat a medium skillet sprayed with nonstick spray over medium-low heat. Pour ¼ cup batter into skillet and cook until surface bubbles. Flip pancake and continue cooking until golden brown.
5. Repeat with remaining batter.

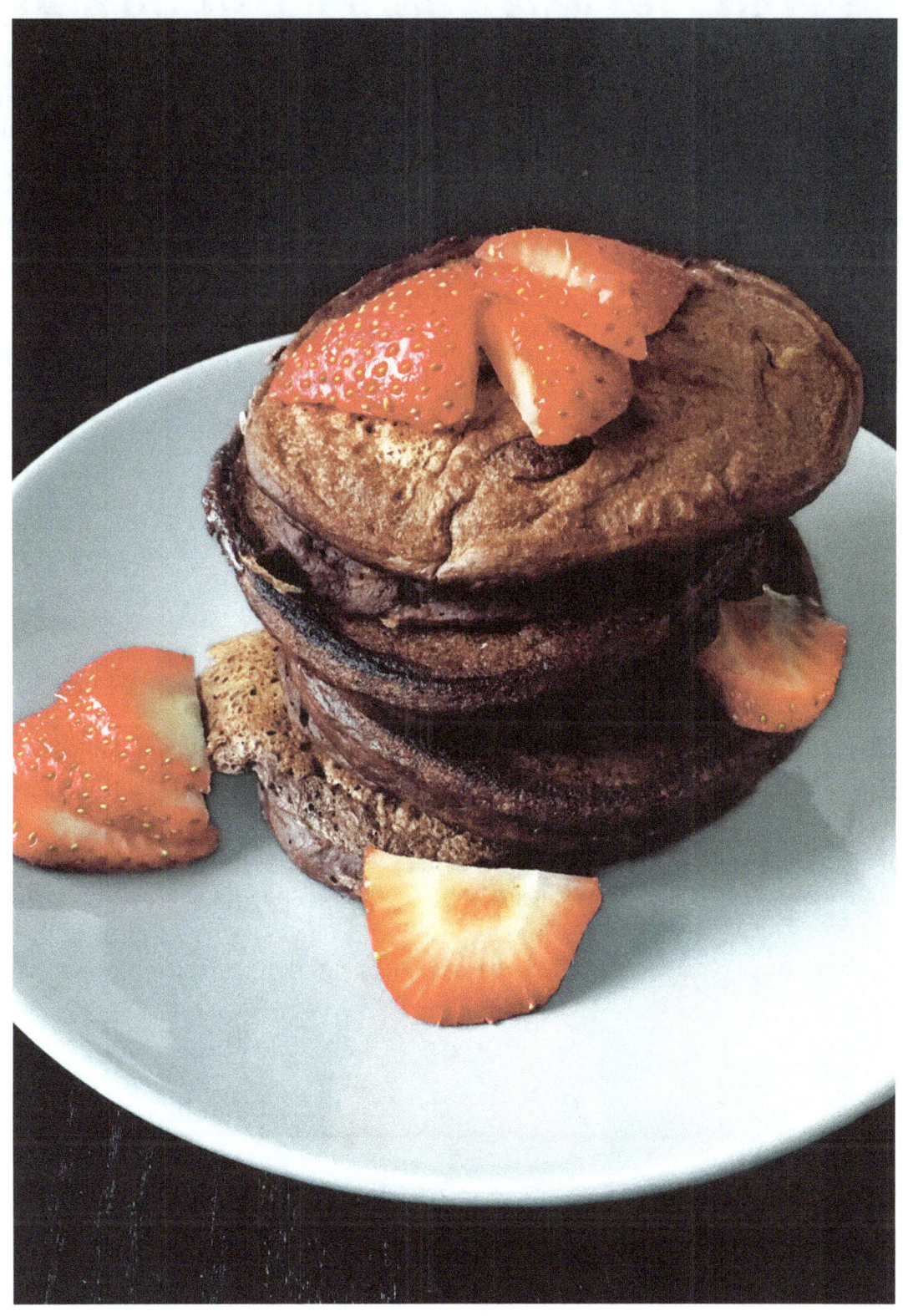

Fruity French Toast Casserole

This recipe is a perfect meal for a weekend morning or a Sunday family brunch gathering. With whole wheat bread and a variety of fruit, it is a healthy breakfast that goes well with a cup of low fat milk to add calcium and vitamin D to start your day!

MAKES 6 SERVINGS

INGREDIENTS

- ½ cup chopped green apple
- 2 teaspoons lemon juice
- 6 slices whole wheat bread, cut into 1-inch pieces
- ¾ cup fresh blueberries
- ½ cup sliced strawberries
- ¼ cup sugar
- ½ cup low fat milk
- 2 whole eggs
- 4 egg whites
- 1 teaspoon vanilla extract

INSTRUCTIONS

1. Preheat oven to 350°F. Prepare an 8-inch square baking dish with nonstick spray and set aside.
2. In a medium bowl, sprinkle apples with lemon juice to prevent browning. Add whole wheat bread, blueberries, and strawberries and mix well.
3. In a medium bowl, mix sugar and milk together until sugar dissolves. Whisk in whole eggs, egg whites, and vanilla extract. Pour wet ingredients over bread and fruit and gently toss to coat. Let stand for 5 minutes and toss again.
4. Place mixture into prepared baking dish. Bake for 40 minutes or until top is browned and center is set.

Intuitive Eating Wisdom

Intuitive Eating Principle 9: Exercise – Feel the Difference

Say no to rigid, bootcamp style exercise and yes to joyful movement. Rather than exercising to burn calories, focus on movement that feels good for your body. Turn your attention to the way your body feels when you exercise: the energy, the freedom, and the empowerment that comes when you move in a way that feels right. Adapt to what suits your needs and feel the difference in how this mental shift feels in your mind and body.

Muffins & Breads

IN THIS CHAPTER

- 253 | Apple Craisin Muffins
- 254 | Cinnamon Raisin Bread
- 256 | Corn Muffins
- 257 | Banana Oatmeal Muffins
- 258 | Pumpkin Muffins
- 260 | Carrot Raisin Muffins
- 261 | Peanut Butter Bran Muffins
- 262 | Zucchini Carrot Bread
- 264 | Blueberry Oat Bran Muffin
- 265 | Walnut Date Bread

Apple Craisin Muffins

Muffins & Breads

Apples, cinnamon, craisins, oh my! These Apple Craisin Muffins are a great addition to breakfast or snack with a burst of flavor in every bite. Eat them right out of the oven or pop them in the toaster later for a yummy treat!

MAKES 12 SERVINGS

INGREDIENTS

- 1 ¼ cup whole wheat flour
- 1 tablespoon baking powder
- ½ teaspoon ground cinnamon
- ½ teaspoon salt
- 2 cups bran flakes cereal
- 1 cup low fat milk
- 2 egg whites
- ½ cup unsweetened applesauce
- 1 apple, cored and finely chopped
- ⅓ cup craisins

INSTRUCTIONS

1. Preheat oven to 400°F. Prepare a muffin pan with nonstick spray and set aside.
2. In a medium bowl, mix whole wheat flour, baking powder, cinnamon and salt.
3. In a separate bowl, combine bran flakes cereal and milk. Let sit for 5 minutes.
4. Beat egg whites in a small bowl. Add applesauce, chopped apple, and craisins. Add to dry ingredients and combine until moist throughout.
5. Spoon batter into muffin pan, filling each cup ⅔ full.
6. Bake for 20 minutes or until golden brown.

Cinnamon Raisin Bread

Indulge in a slice of this bread with breakfast, lunch, or dinner. Applesauce and sweet potato combine for a moist texture, sweet flavor, and extra nutrients in every slice!

MAKES 20 SERVINGS

INGREDIENTS

- ¾ cup all-purpose flour
- ¾ cup whole wheat flour
- 1 ½ teaspoon baking powder
- ½ teaspoon baking soda
- 1 ½ teaspoons ground cinnamon
- ½ teaspoon ground nutmeg
- ½ teaspoon salt
- ½ cup firmly packed light brown sugar
- ¾ cup raisins
- ⅓ cup unsweetened applesauce
- 4 egg whites
- ½ cup low fat milk
- 1 teaspoon vanilla extract
- 1 cup mashed sweet potato

INSTRUCTIONS

1. Preheat oven to 350°F. Prepare two 9 x 5 x 2 ¾-inch loaf pans with nonstick spray.
2. In a medium bowl, sift together flours, baking powder, baking soda, cinnamon, nutmeg, and salt.
3. Stir in brown sugar and raisins; mix well.
4. In a separate bowl, combine applesauce, egg whites, milk, vanilla extract, and sweet potato and mix well.
5. Add wet ingredients to dry ingredients and mix until moist.
6. Evenly divide batter between two pans and bake for 1 hour.

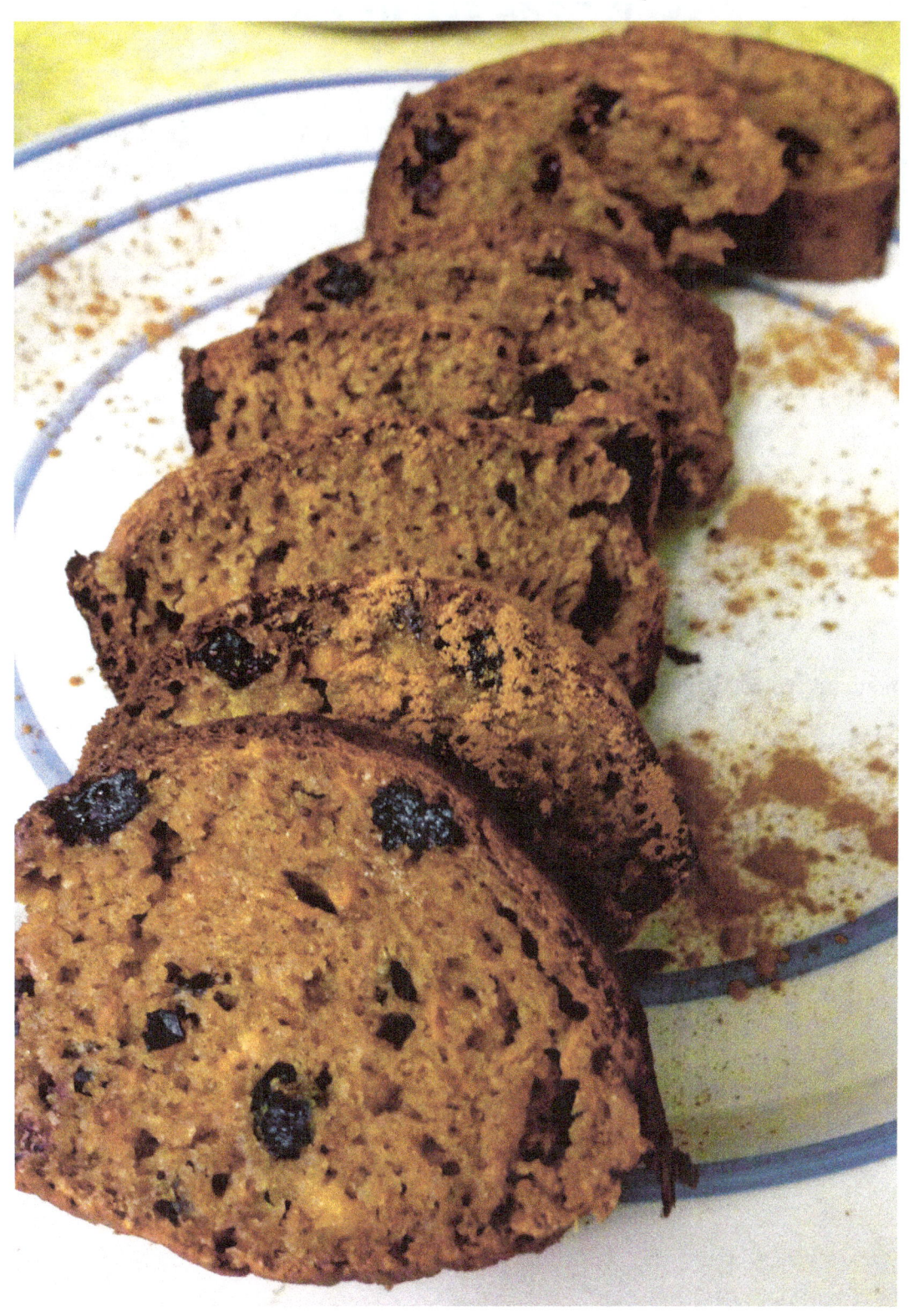

Corn Muffins

Corn muffins are sweet, crumbly, and so delicious, especially when perfectly toasted. Try them with a touch of honey, your favorite spread, or beside hearty vegetable chili.

MAKES 12 SERVINGS

INGREDIENTS

- 1 cup yellow cornmeal
- 1 cup whole wheat flour
- ¼ cup sugar
- ½ teaspoon salt
- 4 teaspoons baking powder
- 1 egg
- 1 cup low fat milk
- ½ teaspoon vanilla extract
- 2 tablespoons unsweetened applesauce

INSTRUCTIONS

1. Preheat oven to 400°F. Prepare a muffin pan with nonstick spray and set aside.
2. In a medium bowl, combine cornmeal, whole wheat flour, sugar, salt, and baking powder.
3. In a separate bowl, beat egg and add milk, vanilla extract, and applesauce. Mix well.
4. Add wet ingredients to dry ingredients and mix until batter becomes moist.
5. Evenly distribute batter into each muffin cup until ⅔ full.
6. Bake for 15 minutes.

Banana Oatmeal Muffins

This is a great muffin recipe to whip up at the beginning of the week for a grab-and-go breakfast on your busy weekday mornings. Nothing gives you lasting energy like bananas and oatmeal to supply your body with fuel to get you through the morning!

MAKES 12 SERVINGS

INGREDIENTS

- 1 cup uncooked old fashioned oatmeal
- ¾ cup whole wheat flour
- ½ cup all-purpose flour
- ½ cup sugar
- 1 tablespoon baking powder
- ½ teaspoon baking soda
- ½ teaspoon salt
- 1 teaspoon ground cinnamon
- 3 medium very ripe bananas, peeled
- 1 cup plain nonfat yogurt
- 2 tablespoons unsweetened applesauce
- ½ cup crushed walnuts (optional)

INSTRUCTIONS

1. Preheat oven to 375°F. Line 12 medium muffin cups with paper liners or spray bottoms with nonstick spray and set aside.
2. In a food processor, process oatmeal until it resembles coarse flour, about 15 seconds.
3. Add flours, sugar, baking powder, baking soda, salt, and cinnamon. Pulse a few times to combine. Transfer mixture to a large mixing bowl.
4. In a medium bowl, mash bananas until coarse consistency. Add yogurt and applesauce and mix well. Combine until smooth.
5. Add wet ingredients to dry ingredients and stir by hand, quickly and lightly, until just mixed. Batter will be thick. Add walnuts if desired.
6. Divide batter evenly between prepared muffin cups. Bake for 20-25 minutes in preheated oven.

Pumpkin Muffins

Pumpkin is a favorite throughout the fall season and these muffins are a perfect way to get fall-festive any time of the year. This recipe combines the harvest flavors of pumpkin, cinnamon, and nutmeg into a warm, tasty treat that your whole family will love!

MAKES 12 SERVINGS

INGREDIENTS

- 1 ½ cups whole wheat flour
- ¼ cup sugar
- 1 teaspoon salt
- 1 teaspoon ground nutmeg
- 1 ½ teaspoons ground cinnamon
- ¾ teaspoon baking powder
- ½ teaspoon baking soda
- 1 cup canned pumpkin puree
- ½ cup unsweetened applesauce
- ½ cup chopped walnuts
- ½ cup raisins

INSTRUCTIONS

1. Preheat oven to 350°F. Prepare a muffin pan with nonstick spray and set aside.
2. In a medium bowl, combine flour, sugar, salt, nutmeg, cinnamon, baking powder, and baking soda; mix well.
3. Add pumpkin puree, applesauce, walnuts, and raisins to mixing bowl and mix well.
4. Evenly divide batter amongst muffin cups until ⅔ full.
5. Bake for 15-18 minutes or until toothpick inserted into center of muffin comes out clean.

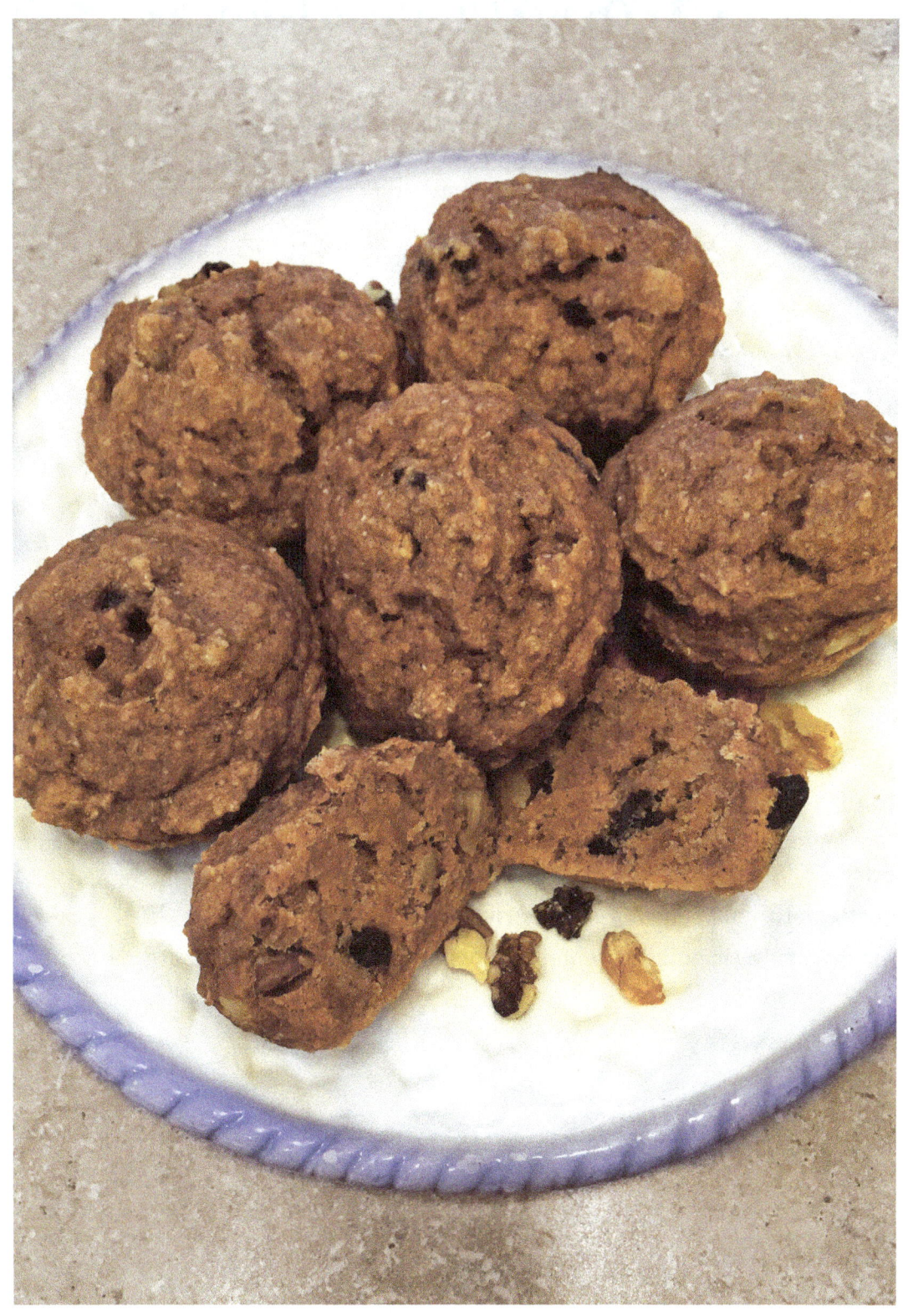

Carrot Raisin Muffins

Get your fill of vegetables in a tasty muffin. These are sweet and moist with a bit of crunchy texture thanks to the grated carrots. Perfect for a nutritious bite any time of day or think outside the box and include them as a side to any meal.

MAKES 12 SERVINGS

INGREDIENTS

- 1 ½ cups whole wheat flour
- ½ cup brown sugar
- 1 teaspoon baking powder
- 1 teaspoon ground cinnamon
- 4 egg whites
- 1 cup low fat milk
- ¼ cup unsweetened applesauce
- ½ teaspoon vanilla extract
- 2 ½ cups grated carrots
- ½ cup raisins

INSTRUCTIONS

1. Preheat oven to 400°F. Prepare a muffin tin with nonstick spray and set aside.
2. In a medium bowl, combine flour, sugar, baking powder, and cinnamon.
3. In a separate bowl, beat egg whites. Mix in milk, applesauce, vanilla extract, grated carrots, and raisins.
4. Add wet ingredients to dry ingredients and stir for about a minute or until batter becomes smooth.
5. Pour batter into muffin tin until each is ⅔ full.
6. Cook in oven for 20 minutes on center rack or until golden brown and toothpick comes out clean.

Muffins & Breads

Peanut Butter Bran Muffins

Peanut butter lovers will go nuts for these muffins! Packed with protein, healthy fats, and fiber, this is a tasty, versatile muffin that can be enjoyed for breakfast, as a snack, or a dessert.

MAKES 12 SERVINGS

INGREDIENTS

- 1 cup bran flakes cereal
- ½ cup low fat milk
- 1 ¼ cup whole wheat flour
- 1 ½ teaspoons baking powder
- ¼ cup sugar
- 1 whole egg, beaten
- 2 egg whites, beaten
- ⅓ cup all-natural peanut butter

INSTRUCTIONS

1. Preheat oven to 375°F. Prepare a muffin pan with nonstick spray and set aside.
2. Combine bran flakes cereal and milk in a bowl. Set aside for 5-6 minutes until bran cereal softens.
3. In a medium bowl, combine flour, baking powder, baking soda, and sugar. Mix well.
4. Add egg, egg whites, peanut butter, and softened bran cereal and mix well.
5. Evenly distribute batter in muffin cups until ⅔ full.
6. Bake for 15-18 minutes or until toothpick inserted into center of muffin comes out clean.

Zucchini Carrot Bread

This bread is perfect for satisfying even the pickiest of eaters. It uses whole vegetables and is chock full of nutrients and flavor. There is a perfect balance of sweetness and is delightfully crunchy. Enjoy alongside a warm cup of tea or a tall glass of milk.

MAKES 20 SERVINGS

INGREDIENTS

- 2 cups all-purpose flour
- 1 cup whole wheat flour
- 2 teaspoons ground cinnamon
- 1 teaspoon baking soda
- ½ teaspoon baking powder
- 1 teaspoon salt
- 4 egg whites
- ½ cup unsweetened applesauce
- 2 medium carrots, peeled and grated
- 2 medium zucchini, peeled and grated
- ½ cup sugar

INSTRUCTIONS

1. Preheat oven to 350°F. Prepare two 9 x 5 x 2 ¾ -inch loaf pans sprayed with nonstick spray and set aside.
2. In a medium bowl, combine flours, cinnamon, baking soda, baking powder, and salt. Mix well.
3. In a separate bowl, combine egg whites, applesauce, grated carrots, grated zucchini, and sugar. Add wet ingredients to dry ingredients and mix well.
4. Pour batter into prepared loaf pans and bake for 1 hour.

Muffins & Breads

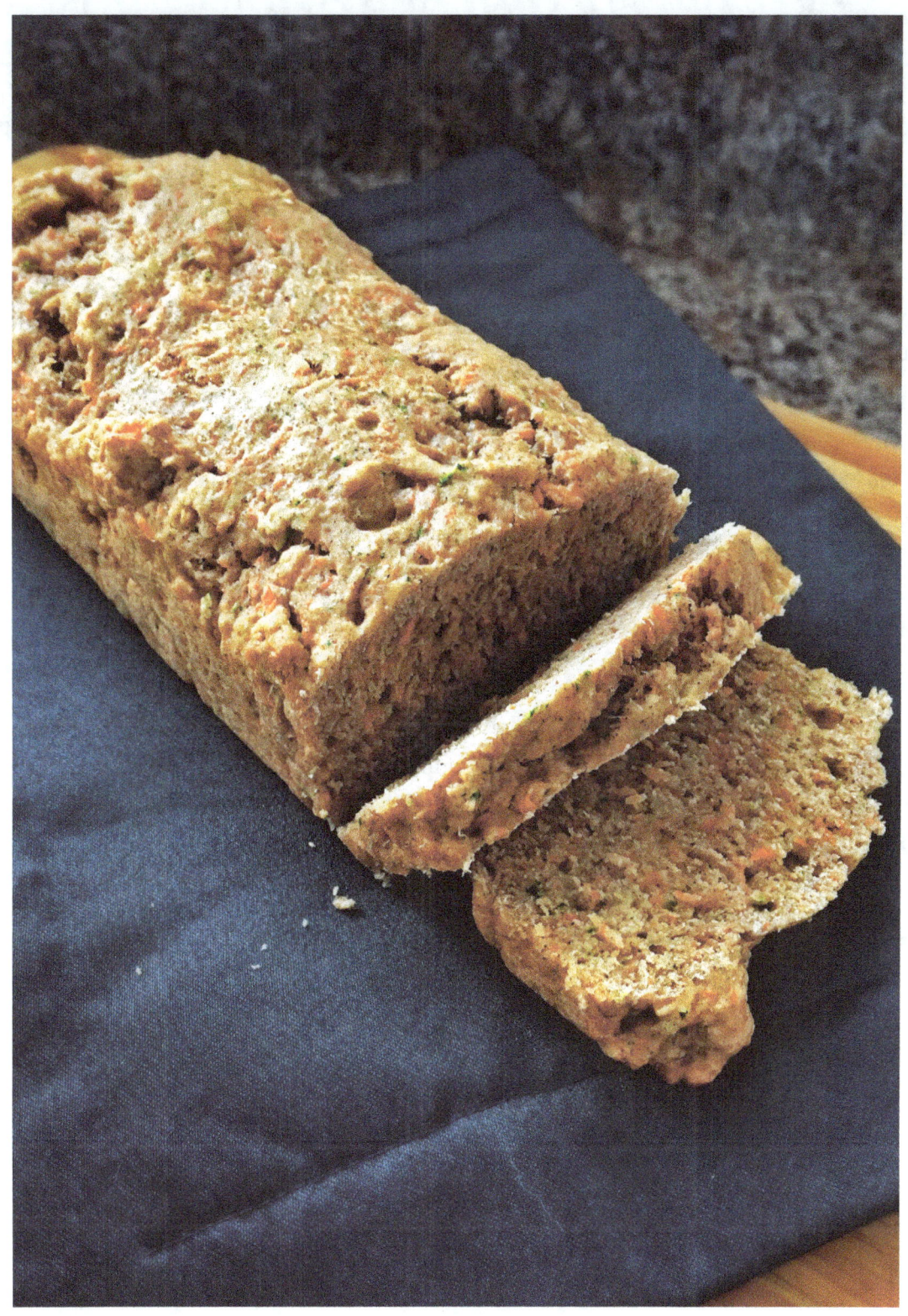

Blueberry Oat Bran Muffins

Wake your family up with the smell of fresh, warm blueberries baking in the oven. These muffins are sweet and full of fiber, vitamins, and minerals to eat alongside breakfast or as a great snack between meals.

MAKES 12 SERVINGS

INGREDIENTS

- ¾ cup uncooked oat bran
- ¾ cup uncooked rolled oats
- 1 ½ cups fresh blueberries
- 1 ½ teaspoons baking powder
- 3 egg whites
- ¼ cup low fat milk
- ½ cup unsweetened applesauce
- 1 teaspoon vanilla extract
- 1 teaspoon ground cinnamon
- 2 tablespoons honey

INSTRUCTIONS

1. Preheat oven to 400°F. Prepare a muffin pan with nonstick spray and set aside.
2. In a medium bowl, combine oat bran, rolled oats, blueberries, and baking powder. Mix well.
3. Beat egg whites in a medium bowl. Add milk, applesauce, vanilla extract, cinnamon, and honey. Mix well.
4. Add wet ingredients to dry ingredients and mix until batter becomes moist.
5. Evenly distribute batter into each muffin cup until ⅔ full.
6. Bake for 20 minutes.

Walnut Date Bread

The sweet flavor of the dates and the crunchiness of the walnuts give this bread a subtly sweet and nutty flavor. It is perfect to eat toasted in the morning as a light breakfast or beside a hot cup of tea!

MAKES 14 SERVINGS

INGREDIENTS

- 2 cups whole wheat flour
- 1 teaspoon baking powder
- ½ teaspoon baking soda
- ¾ teaspoon salt
- ½ cup low fat milk
- ¼ cup sugar
- ¼ cup unsweetened applesauce
- 2 egg whites
- ½ cup chopped dates
- ½ cup chopped walnuts

INSTRUCTIONS

1. Preheat oven to 375°F. Prepare an 8 ½ x 4 ½ x 2 ½-inch loaf pan with nonstick spray and set aside.
2. In a medium bowl, combine flour, baking powder, baking soda, and salt together and mix well.
3. In a separate bowl, combine milk, sugar, applesauce, egg whites, dates, and walnuts and mix well. Add wet ingredients to dry ingredients and stir until batter consistency forms.
4. Pour batter into pan and bake for 45 minutes or until toothpick inserted into center of loaves comes out clean.

Intuitive Eating Wisdom

Intuitive Eating Principle 10: Honor Your Health with Gentle Nutrition

You are in charge of your food decisions. Choose foods that honor your health and taste buds and that feel good in your body. This does not mean every meal needs to be "perfect" but that a consistent effort to be mindful and aware of your food choices will yield long-term benefits. Recognizing that you are in charge of these decisions allows you to be flexible in your habits, respecting your needs as they change.

Desserts

IN THIS CHAPTER
---

271 | Cocoa Peanut Butter Crunch Balls

272 | Quick & Easy Brown Sugar Cookies

274 | Whole Wheat Pie Crust

275 | Strawberry Banana Oat Bars

276 | Double Chocolate Chews

278 | Refreshing Mixed Fruit Kebabs

279 | Sweet Mango Crumble

280 | Cinnamon Coffee Cake

282 | Almond Cookie

283 | Rich Fudge Brownies

284 | Tasty Cheesecake

286 | Light Lemon Cake

287 | Banana Cake

288 | Fruit Cobbler

289 | Cherry Apple Crumble

Dessert

Cocoa Peanut Butter Crunch Balls

Pour yourself a tall glass of milk to enjoy with this peanut butter chocolatey treat! Not only does this dessert combine the delicious flavors of peanut butter and chocolate, but it's also filled with crunchy whole grain flakes for a high fiber indulgence!

MAKES 25 SERVINGS

INGREDIENTS

- 1 cup crushed whole grain cereal flakes
- 2 cups whole wheat flour
- ½ cup unsweetened cocoa powder
- ½ teaspoon salt
- 1 ½ teaspoon baking soda
- 1 ¼ cup unsweetened applesauce
- ¾ cup all-natural crunchy peanut butter
- ½ cup light brown sugar
- 3 egg whites
- 1 ½ teaspoons vanilla extract
- 2 tablespoons chocolate syrup
- ¼ cup dark chocolate chips

INSTRUCTIONS

1. Preheat oven to 375°F. Prepare two baking sheets with nonstick spray and set aside.
2. In a medium bowl, combine crushed cereal, whole wheat flour, cocoa powder, salt, and baking soda.
3. In a large bowl, beat together the applesauce, peanut butter, brown sugar, egg whites, vanilla extract, and chocolate syrup.
4. Stir dry cereal mixture into wet mixture and combine thoroughly. Add chocolate chips and mix well.
5. Drop the batter, by rounded tablespoon, onto the prepared baking sheets and flatten with back of spoon.
6. Cook for approximately 12 minutes or until lightly browned around the edges.

Quick & Easy Brown Sugar Cookies

This recipe yields a perfectly sweet cookie that is high in fiber. Utilizing simple ingredients, these cookies are easy to whip up from your basic kitchen ingredients!

MAKES 14 SERVINGS

INGREDIENTS

- 1 ½ cups coarsely milled oat bran
- 1 cup all-purpose flour
- ½ teaspoon baking soda
- ½ teaspoon salt
- ¼ cup low fat margarine
- ¼ cup canola oil
- ⅓ cup apple juice
- ⅓ cup packed light brown sugar
- 2 egg whites
- 1 teaspoon vanilla extract
- Confectionary sugar, for garnish

INSTRUCTIONS

1. Preheat oven to 400°F. Prepare two baking sheets with nonstick spray and set aside.
2. In a medium bowl, combine oat bran, flour, baking soda, and salt. Mix well.
3. In a separate bowl, mix the margarine and oil together. Add the apple juice, brown sugar, egg whites, and vanilla extract. Beat with electric mixer on medium speed.
4. Add the dry ingredients to wet ingredients and mix well.
5. Drop dough by the teaspoon onto the baking sheet, 2-inches apart.
6. Bake for 8-10 minutes or until golden brown and firm to touch. Cool on a wire rack before serving.
7. Sprinkle confectionary sugar over cookies before serving.

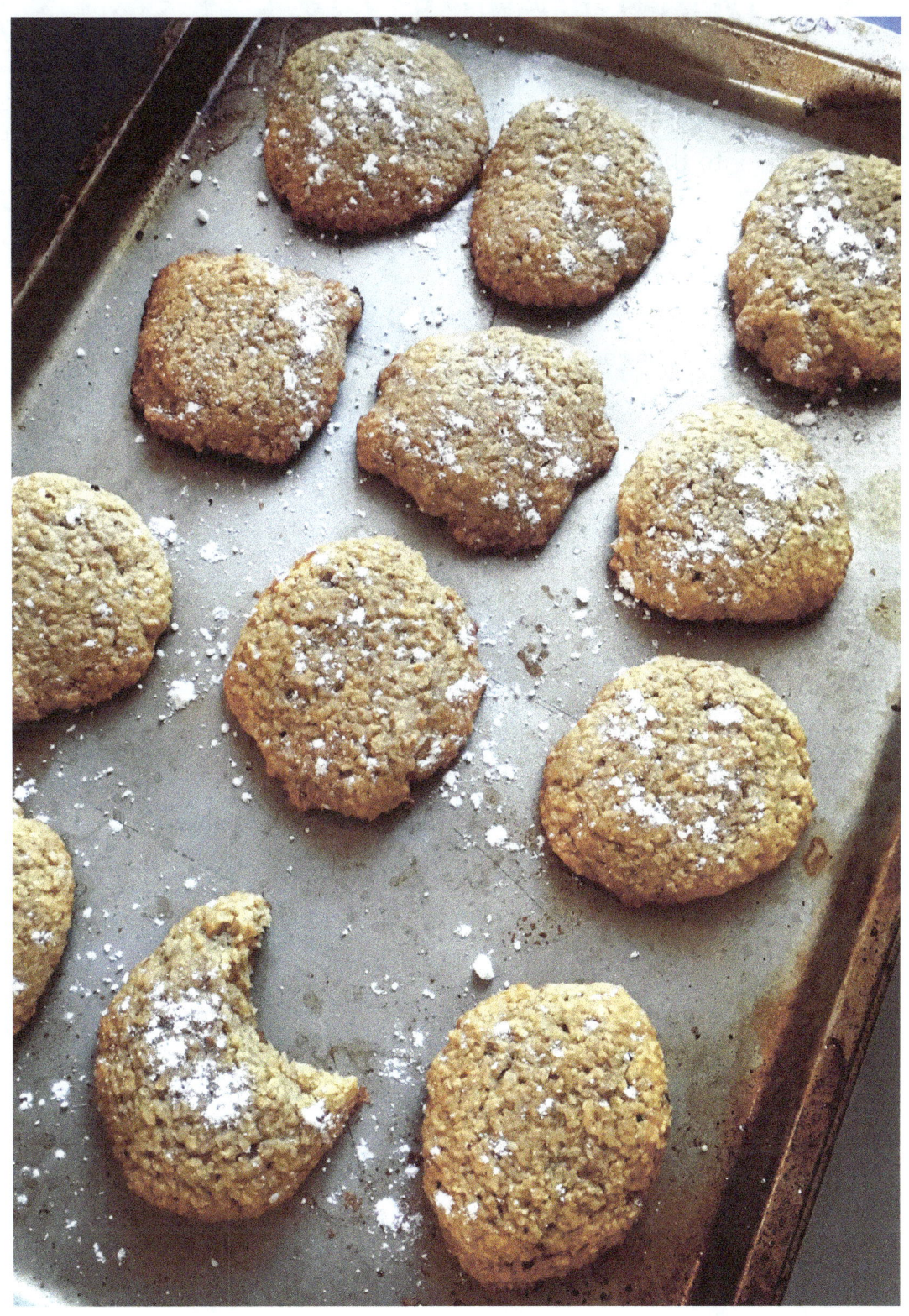

Whole Wheat Pie Crust

Making your own pie crust gives you the chance to customize the ingredients, like using whole wheat flour! There is nothing like a homemade crust to bring your pie to the next level and impress your guests.

MAKES 8 SERVINGS

INGREDIENTS

- ½ cup uncooked quick-cooking oats
- 1 cup whole wheat flour
- 2 tablespoons brown sugar
- ½ teaspoon salt
- 3 tablespoons canola oil
- 7 tablespoons plain soy milk

INSTRUCTIONS

1. Preheat oven to 425°F. Prepare a 9-inch pie pan with nonstick spray and set aside.
2. In a medium bowl, mix together oats, whole wheat flour, brown sugar, and salt.
3. In a small bowl, mix canola oil and soy milk together.
4. Add the oil and soy milk mixture to the dry ingredients until it holds together.
5. Press crust mixture into prepared pan and bake for 8-10 minutes or until lightly golden brown.

Dessert

Strawberry Banana Oat Bars

These bars have just the right amount of sweetness and are high in fiber. They are perfectly crunchy yet chewy at the same time and will satisfy any palate.

MAKES 12 SERVINGS

INGREDIENTS

- 1 ½ cups old-fashioned oats
- ½ cup crushed bran flakes cereal
- 2 teaspoons ground cinnamon
- 1 teaspoon salt
- ¼ cup brown sugar
- 1 banana, mashed
- 1 egg, beaten
- 1 teaspoon vanilla extract
- 1 cup sliced strawberries
- ¼ cup dark chocolate chips

INSTRUCTIONS

1. Preheat oven to 350°F. Prepare an 11 x 7-inch baking dish with nonstick spray and set aside.
2. Place oats on a baking sheet in preheated oven for 7-10 minutes. After 5 minutes, flip oats.
3. In a large bowl, mix toasted oats, crushed bran flakes cereal, cinnamon, salt, and brown sugar.
4. In a smaller bowl, combine the mashed banana, egg, and vanilla extract.
5. Combine the wet ingredients into the dry ingredients and mix well. Gently mix in strawberries and chocolate chips.
6. Pour batter into prepared baking dish. Bake for 25 minutes or until edges are golden brown.
7. Allow to cool for 5 minutes before cutting into bars. Refrigerate if not serving immediately or freeze for later use.

Double Chocolate Chews

Double the chocolate satisfaction with these moist and chewy chocolatey cookies. The Greek yogurt in this recipe makes this yummy dessert a good source of protein, a nutrition surprise you don't expect to find in a delicious chocolate cookie!

MAKES 20 SERVINGS

INGREDIENTS

- 4 tablespoons plain nonfat Greek yogurt
- 2 tablespoons low fat margarine, softened
- ½ cup firmly packed brown sugar
- 1 teaspoon vanilla extract
- 1 cup whole wheat flour
- ½ teaspoon salt
- ½ cup unsweetened cocoa
- 2 tablespoons unsweetened applesauce
- ¼ cup mini chocolate chips

INSTRUCTIONS

1. Preheat oven to 350°F. Prepare a baking sheet with nonstick spray and set aside.
2. In a medium bowl, cream together the Greek yogurt, margarine, and brown sugar.
3. Add vanilla extract and mix well.
4. In a separate bowl, sift together whole wheat flour, salt, and cocoa. Mix dry ingredients into the wet ingredients. Stir in the applesauce and chocolate chips and mix well.
5. Roll 1 tablespoon of dough into a ball and place on baking sheet. Continue with remaining dough, placing balls 2-inches apart. Using the bottom of a glass, gently flatten the balls.
6. Bake for 8 minutes or until slightly puffed and soft to the touch.

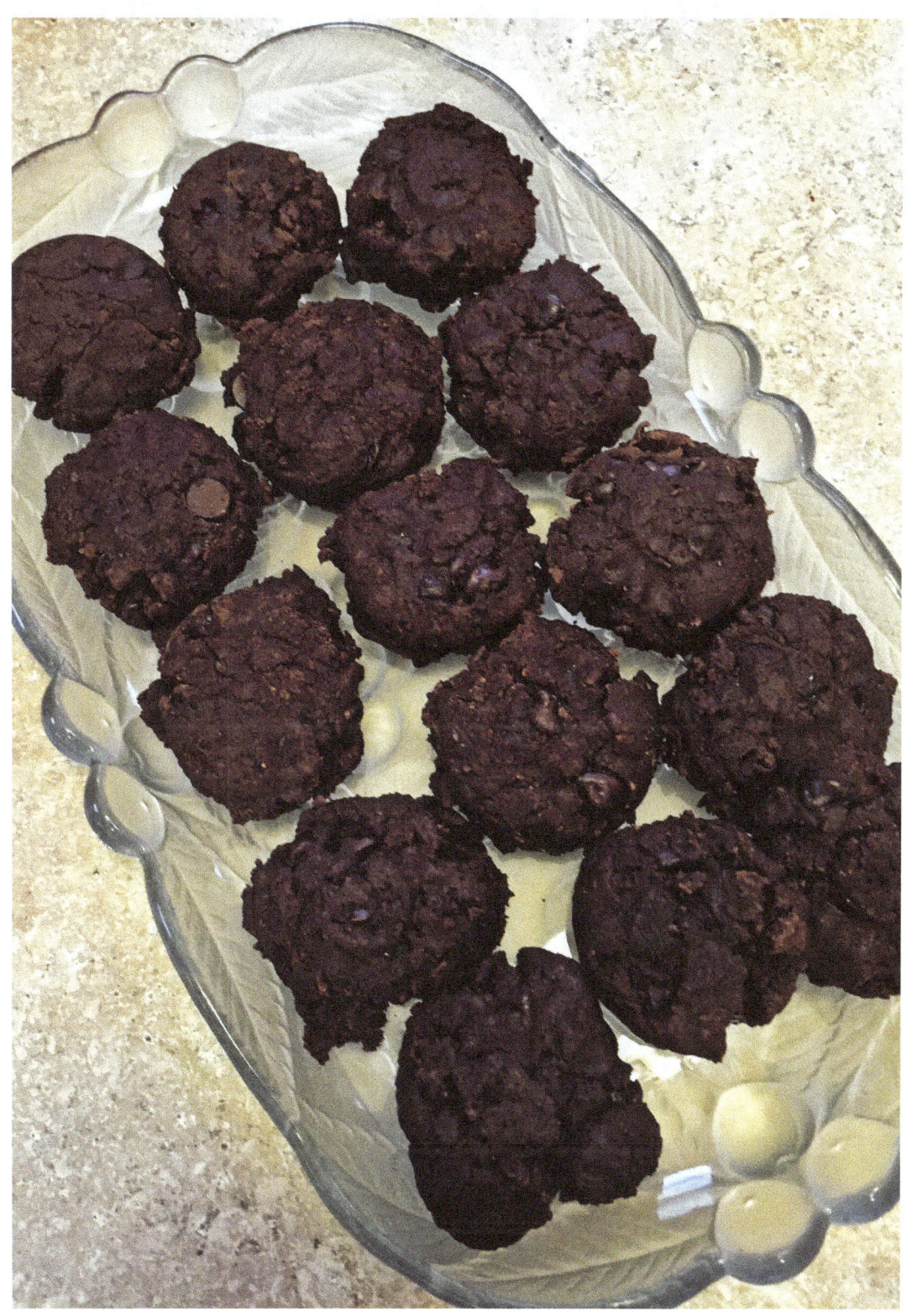

Refreshing Mixed Fruit Kebabs

These sweet kebabs are the perfect refreshment for your summer BBQ. Customize your own fruit kebabs by choosing any fruit combination your heart desires!

MAKES 4 SERVINGS

INGREDIENTS

- ¼ cup fresh lime juice
- ¼ cup apple juice concentrate, thawed
- ¾ teaspoon ground cinnamon
- 2 bananas, sliced into 1 ½ -inch pieces
- 1 mango, peeled, cored and cut into 1 ½-inch pieces
- 1 peach, peeled, cored and cut into 1 ½-inch pieces

INSTRUCTIONS

1. In a medium bowl, combine lime juice, apple juice concentrate, and cinnamon.
2. Toss cut fruit in apple juice mixture and let stand for 5 minutes.
3. Place fruit onto skewers, alternating bananas, mangos, and peaches.
4. Grill for 5-10 minutes or until fruit is soft and lightly browned, turning occasionally.
5. Baste skewers with any additional liquid mixture while grilling.

Dessert

Sweet Mango Crumble

This recipe is a nutritious treat that incorporates the fresh and juicy flavors of mangos and apples. The fruit is topped with a whole wheat crumble mixture containing fiber-filled wheat germ and oats along with crunchy walnuts to provide healthy fats.

MAKES 18 SERVINGS

INGREDIENTS

- ½ cup all-purpose flour, divided
- ¼ cup whole wheat flour
- ½ cup toasted wheat germ
- ¾ cup old-fashioned oats
- ¼ cup brown sugar
- ¼ cup chopped walnuts
- 1 ½ teaspoons ground cinnamon
- 2 tablespoons melted low fat margarine
- 3 medium Golden Delicious apples
- 3 medium Red Delicious apples
- 3 tablespoons lemon juice
- 2 mangos, peeled and chopped

INSTRUCTIONS

1. Preheat oven to 375°F. Prepare a 9 x 13-inch baking dish with nonstick spray and set aside.
2. Mix together ¼ cup all-purpose flour, whole wheat flour, wheat germ, oats, brown sugar, walnuts, and cinnamon in a bowl. Stir in melted margarine and set aside.
3. Core the apples and chop. Spritz with lemon juice and stir. Mix in remaining ¼ cup all-purpose flour; gently fold in mango.
4. Place the apple and mango mixture in prepared baking dish. Sprinkle the flour-oat mixture evenly over the top.
5. Bake for 45 minutes, until the apples are tender.

Cinnamon Coffee Cake

Move over store-bought coffee cake! With ingredients like hearty oats, cinnamon, vanilla, and soy milk, this coffee cake makes for a rich tasting dessert that will bring the taste and aroma of a coffee shop into your kitchen.

MAKES 12 SERVINGS

CRUMBS INGREDIENTS

- ⅓ cup uncooked old fashioned oats
- 2 tablespoons whole wheat flour
- 2 tablespoons sugar
- 1 teaspoon vanilla extract
- 2 tablespoons canola oil

BATTER INGREDIENTS

- 1 ½ cups all-purpose flour
- 2 ½ teaspoons baking powder
- ½ teaspoon salt
- ½ tablespoon ground cinnamon
- ½ cup brown sugar
- ½ cup low fat margarine, softened
- 1 egg
- 1 teaspoon vanilla extract
- ½ cup plain soy milk

INSTRUCTIONS

1. Preheat oven to 350°F. Prepare an 8 x 8-inch baking dish with nonstick spray and set aside.
2. To make the crumbs: In a medium bowl, combine oatmeal, whole wheat flour, sugar, vanilla extract, and oil. Mix until crumbs are formed. Set crumbs aside.
3. To make the batter: In a medium bowl, sift flour, baking powder, salt, and cinnamon. In a separate bowl, cream brown sugar and softened margarine. Add in egg, vanilla extract, and soymilk. Combine wet ingredients into dry ingredients and mix well.
4. Pour batter in prepared pan and sprinkle crumbs on top. Bake for 20-25 minutes or until toothpick inserted into center comes out clean.

Dessert

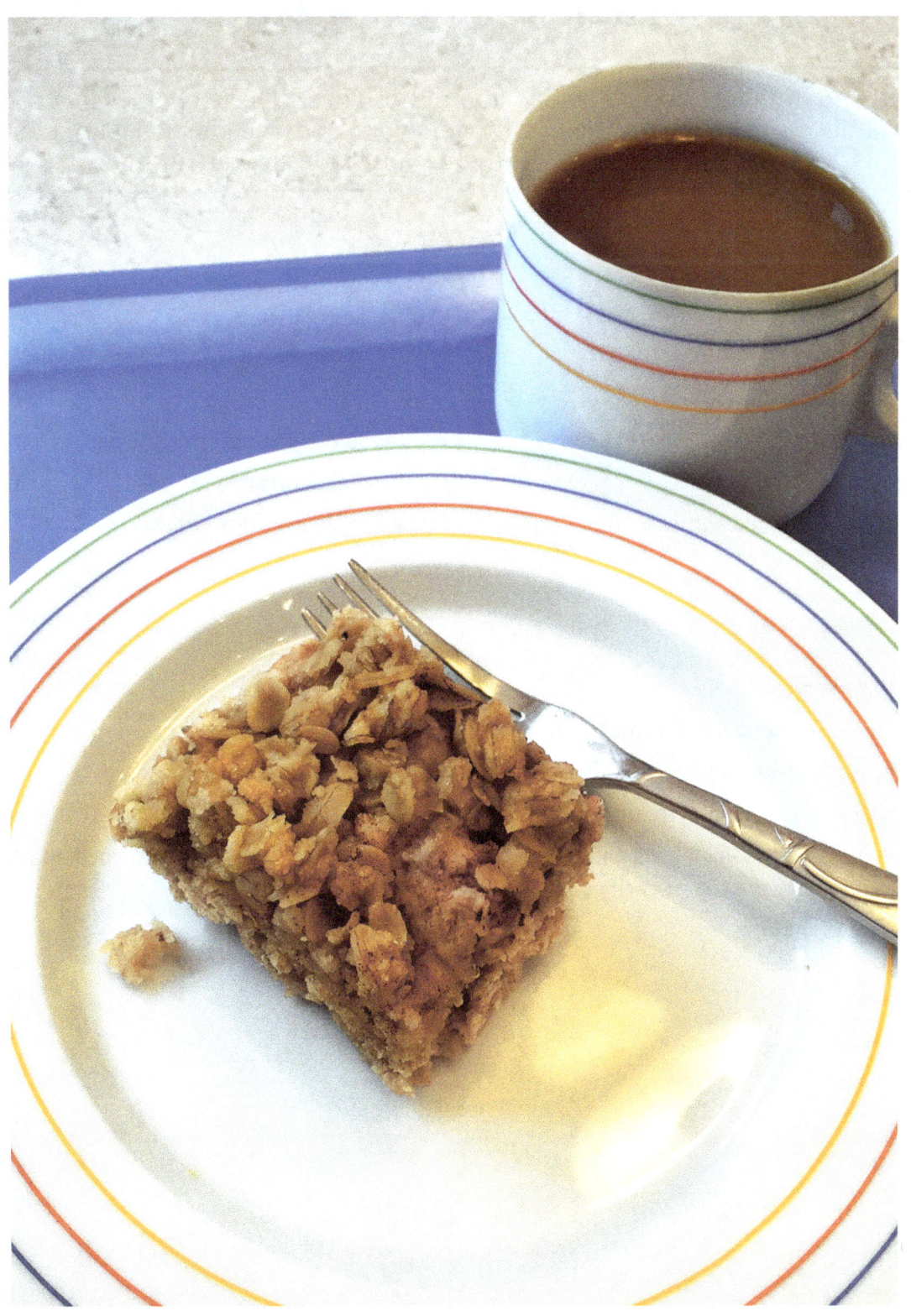

Almond Cookies

You will go nuts for these delicious almond cookies! These cookies incorporate whole almonds to offer you the healthy fats your body needs. Bake up a batch to have a healthy snack ready for your kids to grab-and-go.

MAKES 26 SERVINGS

INGREDIENTS

- 2 ¾ cups all-purpose flour
- ½ teaspoon baking soda
- 1 cup sugar
- ½ teaspoon salt
- ½ cup unsweetened applesauce
- ½ cup canola oil
- 1 teaspoon almond extract
- 1 whole egg, beaten
- 2 tablespoons low fat milk
- 26 whole raw almonds

INSTRUCTIONS

1. Preheat oven to 325°F.
2. In a medium mixing bowl, combine flour, baking soda, sugar and salt.
3. Add applesauce, canola oil, and almond extract to mixture and mix well.
4. Add beaten egg and milk to mixture and mix well.
5. Shape dough into 1-inch balls and place onto ungreased cookie sheet about 1-inch apart. Press an almond onto the top of each cookie.
6. Bake for 15 minutes.

Dessert

Rich Fudge Brownies

What's better than homemade brownies and a tall glass of milk? Enjoy the rich chocolate flavor and chewy texture while you sink your teeth into these moist brownies.

MAKES 18 SERVINGS

INGREDIENTS

- 1 cup all-purpose flour
- ½ cup sugar
- ½ cup brown sugar
- 1 whole egg
- 2 egg whites
- ¼ cup canola oil
- ¼ cup unsweetened applesauce
- ⅓ cup baking cocoa
- 1 ½ teaspoons vanilla extract
- 2 tablespoons semi-sweet chocolate chips

INSTRUCTIONS

1. Preheat oven to 350°F. Prepare a 12 x 8-inch baking dish with nonstick spray and set aside.
2. In a medium mixing bowl, combine flour, sugar, brown sugar, egg, egg whites, oil, applesauce, cocoa, and vanilla extract; mix well.
3. Pour batter in prepared pan. Bake for 20 minutes. Sprinkle with chocolate chips and bake for an additional 10 minutes, or until toothpick inserted near the center comes out clean.

Tasty Cheesecake

This creamy and flavorful cheesecake is out of this world and so simple to make at home. Top with strawberries or add your own favorite topping for a customized treat!

MAKES 8 SERVINGS

INGREDIENTS

- 3 (8-ounce) packages light cream cheese, softened
- ½ cup sugar
- 1 teaspoon vanilla extract
- 1 whole egg
- 4 egg whites
- ½ cup graham cracker crumbs
- Boiling water
- 2 cups sliced fresh strawberries

INSTRUCTIONS

1. Preheat oven to 325°F. Prepare a 9-inch pie plate with nonstick spray and set aside.
2. In a medium bowl, combine cream cheese, sugar, and vanilla extract. Mix with an electric mixer on medium speed until well blended.
3. Add egg and egg whites; mix until blended. Do not overbeat.
4. Sprinkle graham cracker crumbs on bottom of pie plate and pour in cream cheese mixture.
5. Place pie plate into a roasting pan and pour enough boiling water to come 1-inch up from the outside of the pan. Bake on the middle rack of the oven for approximately 45 minutes or until center is almost set.
6. Set aside to cool and refrigerate 3 hours or overnight. Top with strawberry slices.

Dessert

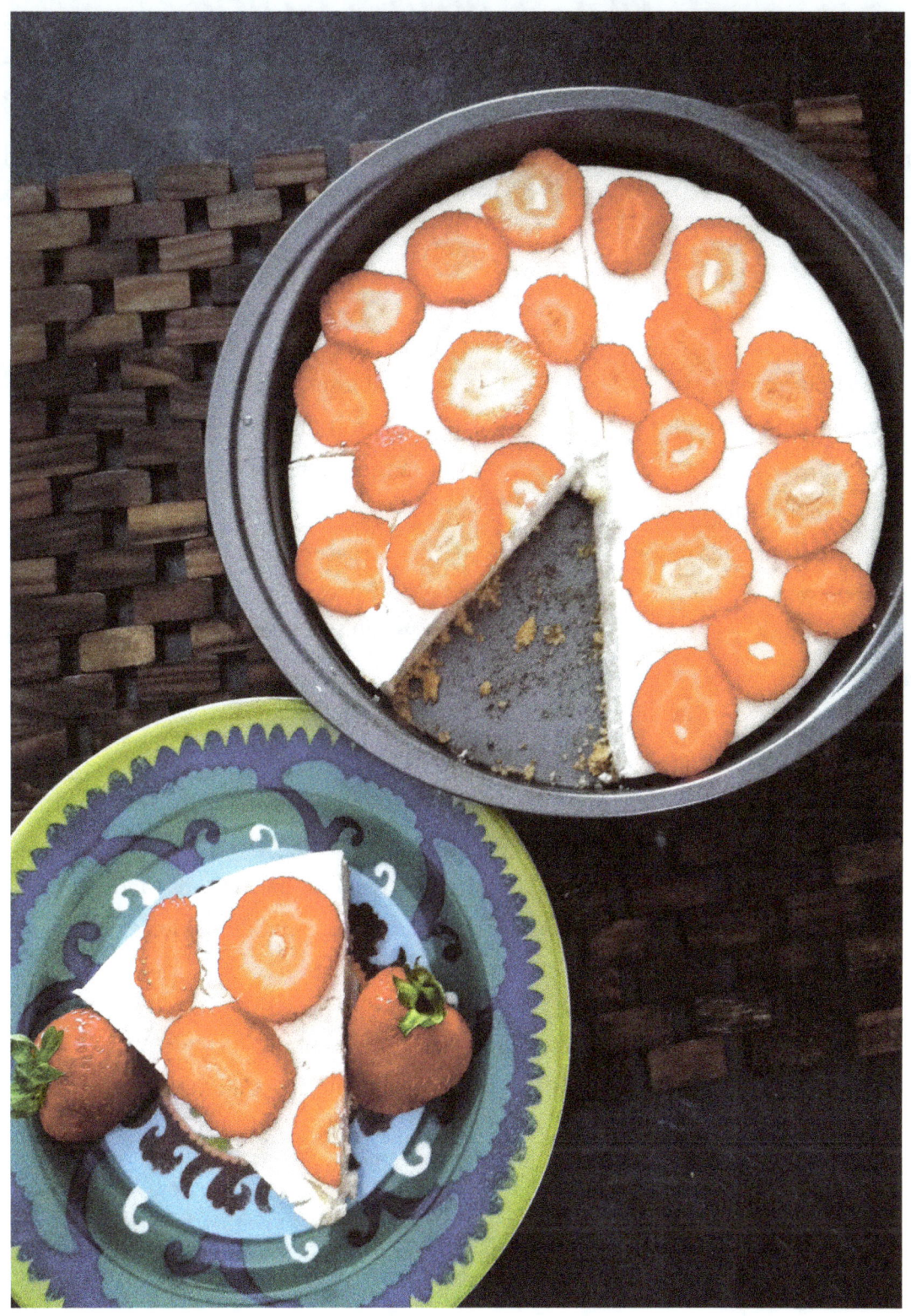

Light Lemon Cake

This recipe makes a perfectly moist lemon cake that is bursting with delicate citrus flavor. The lemon adds a pop of excitement for your taste buds. Top it off with powdered sugar and you are set for any occasion with this simple and elegant dessert.

MAKES 16 SERVINGS

INGREDIENTS

- 1 ¼ cup all-purpose flour
- ¾ cup whole wheat flour
- ½ cup sugar
- 1 teaspoon baking powder
- 1 teaspoon baking soda
- ½ teaspoon salt
- 1 cup low fat milk
- 2 egg whites
- 2 tablespoons canola oil
- 1 ½ grated lemon zest
- 1 teaspoon fresh lemon juice
- 1 teaspoon vanilla extract
- 1 ½ teaspoons confectionery sugar, for garnish
- ¼ cup sliced fresh strawberries, for garnish

INSTRUCTIONS

1. Preheat oven to 350°F. Prepare an 8 x 8-inch baking dish with nonstick spray and set aside.
2. In a large mixing bowl, combine flours, sugar, baking powder, baking soda, and salt.
3. In a separate bowl, stir together milk, egg whites, oil, lemon zest, lemon juice, and vanilla extract.
4. Add wet ingredients to dry ingredients and stir until moist.
5. Pour batter into prepared pan. Bake for approximately 35 minutes.
6. Sift confectionery sugar over cake and top with fresh strawberry slices, if desired.

Dessert

Banana Cake

Wondering what to do with those spotty, ripe bananas? Make a nutritious, moist banana cake, of course! The cinnamon and vanilla combine with the bananas to make a rich, sweet cake that is delicious enough to go icing-free.

MAKES 16 SERVINGS

INGREDIENTS

- 2 cups whole wheat flour
- 1 ½ teaspoons baking soda
- 1 teaspoon baking powder
- ½ teaspoon salt
- 2 egg whites
- ½ cup sugar
- 4 very ripe bananas, mashed
- 1 teaspoon vanilla extract
- ⅓ cup unsweetened applesauce
- 1 teaspoon ground cinnamon

INSTRUCTIONS

1. Preheat oven to 350°F. Prepare a 9-inch Bundt pan with nonstick spray.
2. In a medium bowl, sift flour, baking soda, baking powder, and salt together.
3. In a large bowl, cream together egg whites and sugar.
4. Add the mashed bananas, vanilla extract, applesauce, and cinnamon. Mix well.
5. Gradually stir in the dry ingredients and mix until just blended.
6. Pour batter into prepared Bundt pan and bake for 1 hour.

Fruit Cobbler

Try this cobbler for a tasty way to get an extra serving of fruit into your day. Not only does this recipe yield a fresher, more delicious flavor than store bought fruit pie, it's a great way to use the fruits you already have at home. Peaches, plums, and raspberries combine for a divine cobbler but this recipe can include any fruit you have on hand.

MAKES 8 SERVINGS

INGREDIENTS

- 3 medium peaches, sliced
- 3 medium plums, sliced
- 1 cup fresh raspberries
- ¼ cup sugar, divided
- 1 tablespoon corn starch
- 1 teaspoon lemon juice
- ½ teaspoon ground cinnamon
- 3 sheets graham crackers
- 1 cup all-purpose flour
- 1 ½ teaspoons baking powder
- ½ teaspoon salt
- 3 tablespoons low fat margarine
- 2 teaspoons plain soy milk

INSTRUCTIONS

1. Preheat oven to 350°F.
2. In a saucepan, combine peaches, plums, raspberries, 1 tablespoon sugar, corn starch, lemon juice, and cinnamon. Bring mixture to a boil over medium heat. Cook until mixture thickens, about 1 minute. Remove from heat and transfer mixture to an 8 x 8-inch square baking dish.
3. Place graham crackers in a sealed plastic bag and use fist to crush. In a bowl, combine crushed graham crackers, flour, remaining sugar, baking powder, and salt. Work in margarine with a fork until mixture resembles coarse crumbs.
4. Add soy milk and stir until dry ingredients are evenly moistened.
5. Cover peaches, plums, and raspberry mixture with crumb topping. Bake until topping is brown; approximately 20-25 minutes.

Dessert

Cherry Apple Crumble

Are you looking for an alternative to the classic apple pie? The sweet cherry filling balances the tart apples for a perfect ending to your meal. The soft crumble topping isn't half bad either!

MAKES 10 SERVINGS

INGREDIENTS

- 1 cup all-purpose flour
- 1 ½ cups uncooked old fashioned oatmeal
- ¼ cup sugar
- 1 teaspoon vanilla extract
- ¼ cup canola oil
- 2 egg whites
- 1 teaspoon baking powder
- 3 Granny Smith apples, peeled and cut into small cubes
- 1 (21-ounce) can light cherry filling
- Ground cinnamon, for garnish

INSTRUCTIONS

1. Preheat oven to 350°F. Prepare an 8 x 8-inch pan with nonstick spray and set aside.
2. In a large bowl, combine flour, oatmeal, sugar, vanilla extract, oil, egg whites, and baking powder. Mix until crumbs are formed.
3. Place ⅓ of crumbs on bottom of prepared pan.
4. Top with cubed apples and another ⅓ of the crumbs.
5. Pour lite cherry filling over crumbs. Top with remaining crumbs and sprinkle with cinnamon.
6. Bake uncovered for approximately 1 hour.

Appendix

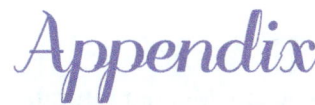

GENTLE NUTRITION FACTS

Soups

AMAZING ARTICHOKE SOUP *page 11*
Makes 5 servings; Serving Size: 1 cup
Calories: 110, Total Fat: 3 gm, Saturated Fat: 0 gm, Monounsaturated Fat: 2 gm, Polyunsaturated Fat: 0 gm, Cholesterol: 0 mg, Protein: 4 gm, Carbohydrate: 18 gm, Dietary Fiber: 4 gm, Sodium: 240 mg

OLD-FASHIONED HEARTY CHICKEN SOUP *page 12*
Makes 8 servings; Serving size: 1 cup
Calories: 330, Total Fat: 21 gm, Saturated Fat: 6 gm, Monounsaturated Fat: 10 gm, Polyunsaturated Fat: 4 gm, Cholesterol: 150 mg, Protein: 29 gm, Carbohydrate: 7 gm, Dietary Fiber: 2 gm, Sodium: 450 mg

ROASTED CHESTNUT SOUP *page 14*
Makes 15 servings; Serving size: 1 cup
Calories: 90, Total Fat: 1 gm, Saturated Fat: 0 gm, Monounsaturated Fat: 0 gm, Polyunsaturated Fat: 0 gm, Cholesterol: 0 mg, Protein: 2 gm, Carbohydrate: 18 gm, Dietary Fiber: 2 gm, Sodium: 140 mg

CHUNKY VEGETABLE SOUP *page 15*
Makes 14 servings; Serving size: 1 cup
Calories: 40, Total Fat: 0 gm, Saturated Fat: 0 mg, Monounsaturated Fat: 0 gm, Polyunsaturated Fat: 0 gm, Cholesterol: 0 mg, Protein: 2 gm, Carbohydrate: 8 gm, Dietary Fiber: 3 gm, Sodium: 90 mg

SWEET & SPICY CARROT SOUP *page 16*
Makes 7 servings; Serving size: 1 cup
Calories: 110, Total Fat: 1 gm, Saturated Fat: 0 gm, Monounsaturated Fat: 0 gm, Polyunsaturated Fat: 0 gm, Cholesterol: 0 mg, Protein: 2 gm, Carbohydrate: 23 gm, Dietary Fiber: 5 gm, Sodium: 310 mg

ZESTY GAZPACHO page 18

Makes 9 servings; Serving size: 1 cup

Calories: 70, Total Fat: 3 gm, Saturated Fat: 0 gm, Monounsaturated Fat: 1.5 gm, Polyunsaturated Fat: 0 gm, Cholesterol: 0 mg, Protein: 2 gm, Carbohydrate: 12 gm, Dietary Fiber: 3 gm, Sodium: 80 mg

CREAM OF BROCCOLI SOUP page 19

Makes 4 servings; Serving size: 1 cup

Calories: 150, Total Fat: 2.5 gm, Saturated Fat: 1 gm, Monounsaturated Fat: 0 gm, Polyunsaturated Fat: 0 gm, Cholesterol: 10 mg, Protein: 12 gm, Carbohydrate: 23 gm, Dietary Fiber: 0 gm, Sodium: 220 mg

MEXICAN SQUASH SOUP page 20

Makes 6 servings; Serving size: 1 cup

Calories: 140, Total Fat: 3 gm, Saturated Fat: 0 gm, Monounsaturated Fat: 2 gm, Polyunsaturated Fat: 0 gm, Cholesterol: 0 mg, Protein: 3 gm, Carbohydrate: 27 gm, Dietary Fiber: 2 gm, Sodium: 200 mg

CREAMY SWEET POTATO SOUP page 22

Makes 15 servings; Serving size: 1 cup

Calories: 80, Total Fat: 1 gm, Saturated Fat: 0 gm, Monounsaturated Fat: 0.5 gm, Polyunsaturated Fat: 0 gm, Cholesterol: 0 mg, Protein: 1 gm, Carbohydrate: 15 gm, Dietary Fiber: 3 gm, Sodium: 190 mg

ONION SOUP page 23

Makes 8 servings; Serving size: 1 cup

Calories: 70, Total Fat: 2 gm, Saturated Fat: 0 gm, Monounsaturated Fat: 1.5 gm, Polyunsaturated Fat: 0 gm, Cholesterol: 0 mg, Protein: 1 gm, Carbohydrate: 10 gm, Dietary Fiber: 2 gm, Sodium: 180 mg

MUSHROOM BARLEY SOUP page 24

Makes 8 servings; Serving size: 1 cup

Calories: 80, Total Fat: 0.5 gm, Saturated Fat: 0 gm, Monounsaturated Fat: 0 gm, Polyunsaturated Fat: 0 gm, Cholesterol: 0 gm, Protein: 4 gm, Carbohydrate: 16 gm, Dietary Fiber: 4 gm, Sodium: 330 mg

Appendix

CORN CHOWDER *page 26*

Makes 5 servings; Serving size: 1 cup

Calories: 180, Total Fat: 5 gm, Saturated Fat: 3 gm, Monounsaturated Fat: 1.5 gm, Polyunsaturated Fat: 0.5 gm, Cholesterol: 15 mg, Protein: 9 gm, Carbohydrate: 29 gm, Dietary Fiber: 2 gm, Sodium: 590 mg

PASTA FAGIOLI SOUP *page 27*

Makes 12 servings; Serving size: 1 cup

Calories: 110, Total Fat: 0.5 gm, Saturated Fat: 0 gm, Monounsaturated Fat: 0 gm, Polyunsaturated Fat: 0 gm, Cholesterol: 0 mg, Protein: 4 gm, Carbohydrate: 19 gm, Dietary Fiber: 5 gm, Sodium: 125 mg

CREAMY TOMATO SOUP WITH COUSCOUS *page 28*

Makes 10 servings; Serving size: 1 cup

Calories: 130, Total Fat: 3 gm, Saturated Fat: 0 gm, Monounsaturated Fat: 1.5 gm, Polyunsaturated Fat: 1 gm, Cholesterol: 0 mg, Protein: 5 gm, Carbohydrate: 21 gm, Dietary Fiber: 3 gm, Sodium: 180 mg

STRAWBERRIES & CRÈME SOUP *page 29*

Makes 5 servings; Serving size: 1 cup

Calories: 110, Total Fat: 0.5 gm, Saturated Fat: 0 gm, Monounsaturated Fat: 0 gm, Polyunsaturated Fat: 0 gm, Cholesterol: 0 gm, Protein: 7 gm, Carbohydrate: 20 gm, Dietary Fiber: 2 gm, Sodium: 75 mg

Salads

COLORFUL HEALTH SALAD *page 35*

Makes 6 servings; Serving size: ½ cup

Calories: 45, Total Fat: 2 gm, Saturated Fat: 0 gm, Monounsaturated Fat: 0 gm, Polyunsaturated Fat: 1 gm, Cholesterol: 0 mg, Protein: <1 gm, Carbohydrate: 6 gm, Dietary Fiber: 1 gm, Sodium: 115 mg

BLACK BEAN & WILD RICE ROMAINE SALAD *page 36*

Makes 12 servings; Serving size: 1 cup

Calories: 200, Total Fat: 10 gm, Saturated Fat: 6 gm, Monounsaturated Fat: 2 gm, Polyunsaturated Fat: 0.5 gm, Cholesterol: 35 mg, Protein: 10 gm, Carbohydrate: 17 gm, Dietary Fiber: 3 gm, Sodium: 370 mg

OUTRAGEOUS CAESAR SALAD *page 38*

Makes 10 servings; Serving size: 1 cup

Calories: 60, Total Fat: 2 gm, Saturated Fat: 1 gm, Monounsaturated Fat: 0.5 gm, Polyunsaturated Fat: 0.5 gm, Cholesterol: <5 gm, Protein: 3 gm, Carbohydrate: 9 gm, Dietary Fiber: 3 gm, Sodium: 180 mg

MIXED GREENS & MANGO SALAD *page 39*

Makes 10 servings; Serving size: 1 cup

Calories: 70, Total Fat: 5 gm, Saturated Fat: 0.5 gm, Monounsaturated Fat: 3.5 gm, Polyunsaturated Fat: 0.5 gm, Cholesterol: 0 mg, Protein: <1 gm, Carbohydrate: 7 gm, Dietary Fiber: 2 gm, Sodium: 10 mg

CHERRY CHILI PEPPER SALAD *page 40*

Makes 7 servings; Serving size: 1 cup

Calories: 50, Total Fat: 1 gm, Saturated Fat: 0 gm, Monounsaturated Fat: 1 gm, Polyunsaturated Fat: 0 gm, Cholesterol: 0 mg, Protein: 1 gm, Carbohydrate: 9 gm, Dietary Fiber: 2 gm, Sodium: 50 mg

PICKLED GREEN BEAN SALAD *page 42*

Makes 4 servings; Serving size: ½ cup

Calories: 25, Total Fat: 0 gm, Saturated Fat: 0 gm, Monounsaturated Fat: 0 gm, Polyunsaturated Fat: 0 gm, Cholesterol: 0 mg, Protein: 2 gm, Carbohydrate: 4 gm, Dietary Fiber: 0 gm, Sodium: 75 mg

JICAMA SALAD *page 43*

Makes 7 servings; Serving size: ½ cup

Calories: 65, Total Fat: 4 gm, Saturated Fat: 0.5 gm, Monounsaturated Fat: 3 gm, Polyunsaturated Fat: 0 gm, Cholesterol: 0 mg, Protein: <1 gm, Carbohydrate: 7 gm, Dietary Fiber: 2 gm, Sodium: 90 mg

MARINATED VEGETABLE MEDLEY *page 44*

Makes 12 servings; Serving size: 1 cup

Calories: 60, Total Fat: 1 gm, Saturated Fat: 0 gm, Monounsaturated Fat: 0.5 gm, Polyunsaturated Fat: 0 gm, Cholesterol: 0 mg, Protein: 3 gm, Carbohydrate: 11 gm, Dietary Fiber: 5 gm, Sodium: 40 mg

Appendix

ITALIAN HERB TOMATO SALAD *page 46*

Makes 4 servings; Serving size: ½ cup

Calories: 15, Total Fat: 0 gm, Saturated Fat: 0 gm, Monounsaturated Fat: 0 gm, Polyunsaturated Fat: 0 gm, Cholesterol: 0 mg, Protein: <1 gm, Carbohydrate: 3 gm, Dietary Fiber: <1 gm, Sodium: 0 mg

CHICKPEA SALAD *page 47*

Makes 6 servings; Serving size: ¾ cup

Calories: 140, Total Fat: 4.5 gm, Saturated Fat: 0.5 gm, Monounsaturated Fat: 2.5 gm, Polyunsaturated Fat: 1 gm, Cholesterol: 0 mg, Protein: 6 gm, Carbohydrate: 21 gm, Dietary Fiber: 7 gm, Sodium: 270 mg

MIXED GREENS CITRUS BERRY SALAD *page 48*

Makes 6 servings; Serving size: 1 cup

Calories: 90, Total Fat: 6 gm, Saturated Fat: 1 gm, Monounsaturated Fat: 3.5 gm, Polyunsaturated Fat: 1.5 gm, Cholesterol: 0 mg, Protein: 1 gm, Carbohydrate: 10 gm, Dietary Fiber: 2 gm, Sodium: 10 mg

SHREDDED CARROT & RAISIN SALAD *page 50*

Makes 6 servings; Serving size: ½ cup

Calories: 120, Total Fat: 0 gm, Saturated Fat: 0 gm, Monounsaturated Fat: 0 gm, Polyunsaturated Fat: 0 gm, Cholesterol: 0 mg, Protein: 2 gm, Carbohydrate: 27 gm, Dietary Fiber: 4 gm, Sodium: 75 mg

Dips & Dressings

CLASSIC MARINADE *page 55*

Makes 5 servings; Serving size: 2 tablespoons

Calories: 40, Total Fat: 3 gm, Saturated Fat: 0 gm, Monounsaturated Fat: 2 gm, Polyunsaturated Fat: 0 gm, Cholesterol: 0 mg, Protein: 0 gm, Carbohydrate: 2 gm, Dietary Fiber: 0 gm, Sodium: 0 mg

YOGURT DILL SAUCE *page 56*

Makes 4 servings; Serving size: 2 tablespoons

Calories: 45, Total Fat: 3.5 gm, Saturated Fat: .5 gm, Monounsaturated Fat: 1 gm, Polyunsaturated Fat: 2 gm, Cholesterol: <5 mg, Protein: <1 gm, Carbohydrate: 3 gm, Dietary Fiber: 0 gm, Sodium: 280 mg

BALSAMIC VINAIGRETTE *page 58*

Makes 5 servings; Serving size: 2 tablespoons

Calories: 70, Total Fat: 5 gm, Saturated Fat: 1 gm, Monounsaturated Fat: 4 gm, Polyunsaturated Fat: 0.5 gm, Cholesterol: 0 mg, Protein: 0 gm, Carbohydrate: 4 gm, Dietary Fiber: 0 gm, Sodium: 135 mg

CAESAR DRESSING *page 59*

Makes 6 servings; Serving size: 2 tablespoons

Calories: 15, Total Fat: 0.5 gm, Saturated Fat: 0 gm, Monounsaturated Fat: 0 gm, Polyunsaturated Fat: 0 gm, Cholesterol: <5 mg, Protein: <1 gm, Carbohydrate: 2 gm, Dietary Fiber: 0 gm, Sodium: 110 mg

SPINACH ARTICHOKE DIP *page 60*

Makes 26 servings; Serving size: ¼ cup

Calories: 50, Total Fat: 2 gm, Saturated Fat: 0 gm, Monounsaturated Fat: 0 gm, Polyunsaturated Fat: 1 gm, Cholesterol: 2 mg, Protein: 3 gm, Carbohydrate: 7 gm, Dietary Fiber: 3 gm, Sodium: 260 mg

HONEY MUSTARD DRESSING *page 62*

Makes 12 servings; Serving size: 1 tablespoon

Calories: 60, Total Fat: 2.5 gm, Saturated Fat: 0 gm, Monounsaturated Fat: 1.5 gm, Polyunsaturated Fat: 0 gm, Cholesterol: 0 mg, Protein: 0 gm, Carbohydrate: 10 gm, Dietary Fiber: 0 gm, Sodium: 15 mg

TOFU-AVOCADO DIP *page 63*

Makes 8 servings; Serving size: 2 tablespoons

Calories: 50, Total Fat: 3.5 gm, Saturated Fat: 1 gm, Monounsaturated Fat: 2 gm, Polyunsaturated Fat: 1 gm, Cholesterol: 0 mg, Protein: 2 gm, Carbohydrate: 3 gm, Dietary Fiber: 1 gm, Sodium: 160 mg

PINEAPPLE SALSA *page 64*

Makes 5 servings; Serving size: ¼ cup

Calories: 30, Total Fat: 0 gm, Saturated Fat: 0 gm, Monounsaturated Fat: 0 gm, Polyunsaturated Fat: 0 gm, Cholesterol: 0 mg, Protein: 0 gm, Carbohydrate: 9 gm, Dietary Fiber: <1 gm, Sodium: 0 mg

Appendix

HUMMUS page 66

Makes 24 servings; Serving size: 2 tablespoons

Calories: 35, Total Fat: 1 gm, Saturated Fat: 0 gm, Monounsaturated Fat: 0 gm, Polyunsaturated Fat: 0 gm, Cholesterol: 0 mg, Protein: 2 gm, Carbohydrate: 6 gm, Dietary Fiber: 1 gm, Sodium: 110 mg

SPICY SALSA page 67

Makes 6 servings; Serving size: 2 tablespoons

Calories: 25, Total Fat: 0 gm, Saturated Fat: 0 gm, Monounsaturated Fat: 0 gm, Polyunsaturated Fat: 0 gm, Cholesterol: 0 mg, Protein: 1 gm, Carbohydrate: 5 gm, Dietary Fiber: 1 gm, Sodium: 10 mg

Hot Sides

VERY MOIST STUFFING page 73

Makes 8 servings; Serving size: ½ cup

Calories: 160, Total Fat: 1.5 gm, Saturated Fat: 0 gm, Monounsaturated Fat: 0 gm, Polyunsaturated Fat: 1 gm, Cholesterol: 0 mg, Protein: 6 gm, Carbohydrate: 30 gm, Dietary Fiber: 3 gm, Sodium: 280 mg

SAUTÉED SPINACH & LEEKS page 74

Makes 6 servings; Serving size: 1 cup

Calories: 110, Total Fat: 6 gm, Saturated Fat: 0.5 gm, Monounsaturated Fat: 2.5 gm, Polyunsaturated Fat: 2 gm, Cholesterol: 0 mg, Protein: 5 gm, Carbohydrate: 9 gm, Dietary Fiber: 4 gm, Sodium: 170 mg

GARDEN VEGETABLE PACKET page 75

Makes 12 servings; Serving size: ½ cup

Calories: 10, Total Fat: 0 gm, Saturated Fat: 0 gm, Monounsaturated Fat: 0 gm, Polyunsaturated Fat: 0 gm, Cholesterol: 0 mg, Protein: <1 gm, Carbohydrate: 2 gm, Dietary Fiber: 0 gm, Sodium: 105 mg

CRUNCHY BRUSSELS SPROUTS page 76

Makes 6 servings; Serving size: 1 cup

Calories: 70, Total Fat: 2.5 gm, Saturated Fat: 0 gm, Monounsaturated Fat: 1.5 gm, Polyunsaturated Fat: 0 gm, Cholesterol: 0 mg, Protein: 4 gm, Carbohydrate: 10 gm, Dietary Fiber: 4 gm, Sodium: 320 mg

ROASTED VEGETABLE SALAD WITH BASIL VINAIGRETTE page 78

Makes 6 servings; Serving size: 1 cup

Calories: 130, Total Fat: 0 gm, Saturated Fat: 0 gm, Monounsaturated Fat: 0 gm, Polyunsaturated Fat: 0 gm, Cholesterol: 0 mg, Protein: 4 gm, Carbohydrate: 30 gm, Dietary Fiber: 5 gm, Sodium: 40 mg

BROCCOLI SOUFFLÉ page 79

Makes 12 servings; Serving size: 1 piece

Calories: 50, Total Fat: 2 gm, Saturated Fat: 0 gm, Monounsaturated Fat: .5 gm, Polyunsaturated Fat: 1 gm, Cholesterol: 15 mg, Protein: 4 gm, Carbohydrate: 5 gm, Dietary Fiber: 0 gm, Sodium: 170 mg

ASPARAGUS WITH MUSTARD VINAIGRETTE page 80

Makes 8 servings; Serving size: 4 spears

Calories: 45, Total Fat: 3.5 gm, Saturated Fat: 0 gm, Monounsaturated Fat: 2.5 gm, Polyunsaturated Fat: 0 gm, Cholesterol: 0 mg, Protein: 1 gm, Carbohydrate: 3 gm, Dietary Fiber: 1 gm, Sodium: 90 mg

STUFFED GRAPE LEAVES page 82

Makes 7 servings; Serving size: 2 pieces

Calories: 120, Total Fat: 3 gm, Saturated Fat: 0 gm, Monounsaturated Fat: 1.5 gm, Polyunsaturated Fat: 0 gm, Cholesterol: 0 mg, Protein: 3 gm, Carbohydrate: 23 gm, Dietary Fiber: 4 gm, Sodium: 20 mg

RAISIN & CRAISIN POTATO MOUNDS page 83

Makes 12 servings; Serving size: 2 pieces

Calories: 60, Total Fat: 1 gm, Saturated Fat: 0 gm, Monounsaturated Fat: 1 gm, Polyunsaturated Fat: 0 gm, Cholesterol: 0 mg, Protein: <1 gm, Carbohydrate: 12 gm, Dietary Fiber: 1 gm, Sodium: 30 mg

PORTOBELLO MUSHROOM SAUTÉ page 84

Makes 8 servings; Serving size: 1 cup

Calories: 60, Total Fat: 4 gm, Saturated Fat: 1 gm, Monounsaturated Fat: 2.5 gm, Polyunsaturated Fat: 0.5 gm, Cholesterol: 0 mg, Protein: 2 gm, Carbohydrate: 5 gm, Dietary Fiber: 2 gm, Sodium: 35 mg

Appendix

BAKED SWEET POTATO FRIES page 86
Makes 5 servings; Serving size: 3 ounces
Calories: 90, Total Fat: 1.5 gm, Saturated Fat: 0 gm, Monounsaturated Fat: 1 gm, Polyunsaturated Fat: 0 gm, Cholesterol: 0 mg, Protein: 1 gm, Carbohydrate: 18 gm, Dietary Fiber: 3 gm, Sodium: 50 mg

STUFFED POTATO SKINS page 87
Makes 12 servings; Serving size: 1 piece
Calories: 120, Total Fat: 1.5 gm, Saturated Fat: 0 gm, Monounsaturated Fat: 1 gm, Polyunsaturated Fat: 0 gm, Cholesterol: 0 mg, Protein: 5 gm, Carbohydrate: 21 gm, Dietary Fiber: 4 gm, Sodium: 55 mg

MOCK STUFFED DERMA page 88
Makes 12 servings; Serving size: 1 slice
Calories: 110, Total Fat: 4.5 gm, Saturated Fat: 0 gm, Monounsaturated Fat: 2 gm, Polyunsaturated Fat: 1.5 gm, Cholesterol: 0 mg, Protein: 2 gm, Carbohydrate: 16 gm, Dietary Fiber: <1 gm, Sodium: 350 mg

VIBRANT MASHED POTATOES page 90
Makes 12 servings; Serving size: ½ cup
Calories: 100 gm, Total Fat: 1 gm, Saturated Fat: 0 gm, Monounsaturated Fat: 1 gm, Polyunsaturated Fat: 0 gm, Cholesterol: 0 mg, Protein: 3 gm, Carbohydrate: 18 gm, Dietary Fiber: 3 gm, Sodium: 80 mg

BROWN RICE BAKE page 91
Makes 8 servings; Serving size: ½ cup
Calories: 110, Total Fat: 1 gm, Saturated Fat: 0 gm, Monounsaturated Fat: 0.5 gm, Polyunsaturated Fat: 0 gm, Cholesterol: 0 mg, Protein: 2 gm, Carbohydrate: 22 gm, Dietary Fiber: 2 gm, Sodium: 5 mg

GINGER CARAWAY CARROTS page 92
Makes 8 servings; Serving size: 2 carrots
Calories: 50, Total Fat: 2 gm, Saturated Fat: 0 gm, Monounsaturated Fat: 1 gm, Polyunsaturated Fat: 0 gm, Cholesterol: 0 mg, Protein: <1 gm, Carbohydrate: 9 gm, Dietary Fiber: 2 gm, Sodium: 60 mg

COUSCOUS SALAD WITH TOMATOES & ROASTED RED PEPPER *page 94*

Makes 8 servings; Serving size: ½ cup

Calories: 110, Total Fat: 2.5 gm, Saturated Fat: 0 gm, Monounsaturated Fat: 1.5 gm, Polyunsaturated Fat: 0 gm, Cholesterol: 0 mg, Protein: 4 gm, Carbohydrate: 22 gm, Dietary Fiber: 3 gm, Sodium: 160

SPANISH RICE *page 95*

Makes 8 servings; Serving size: ½ cup

Calories: 120, Total Fat: 1.5 gm, Saturated Fat: 0 gm, Monounsaturated Fat: 0.5 gm, Polyunsaturated Fat: 0 gm, Cholesterol: 0 mg, Protein: 3 gm, Carbohydrate: 24 gm, Dietary Fiber: 2 gm, Sodium: 300 mg

PENNE PASTA WITH SPINACH & RED KIDNEY BEANS *page 96*

Makes 8 servings; Serving size: 1 cup

Calories: 210, Total Fat: 4 gm, Saturated Fat: 1 gm, Monounsaturated Fat: 1 gm, Polyunsaturated Fat: 0 gm, Cholesterol: 10 mg, Protein: 13 gm, Carbohydrate: 33 gm, Dietary Fiber: 8 gm, Sodium: 250 mg

BARLEY VEGETABLE MEDLEY *page 98*

Makes 12 servings; Serving size: ½ cup

Calories: 80, Total Fat: 0.5 gm, Saturated Fat: 0 gm, Monounsaturated Fat: 0 gm, Polyunsaturated Fat: 0 gm, Cholesterol: 0 mg, Protein: 3 gm, Carbohydrate: 17 gm, Dietary Fiber: 3 gm, Sodium: 115 mg

CURRIED BROWN RICE SALAD WITH GREEN BEANS *page 99*

Makes 12 servings; Serving size: ½ cup

Calories: 80, Total Fat: 1.5 gm, Saturated Fat: 0 gm, Monounsaturated Fat: 1 gm, Polyunsaturated Fat: 0 gm, Cholesterol: 0 mg, Protein: 2 gm, Carbohydrate: 14 gm, Dietary Fiber: 1 gm, Sodium: 220 mg

TOMATO MUSHROOM BARLEY RISOTTO *page 100*

Makes 8 servings; Serving size: ¾ cup

Calories: 180, Total Fat: 2.5 gm, Saturated Fat: 0 gm, Monounsaturated Fat: 1.5 gm, Polyunsaturated Fat: 0 gm, Cholesterol: 0 mg, Protein: 5 gm, Carbohydrate: 35 gm, Dietary Fiber: 8 gm, Sodium: 220 mg

Appendix

Cold Sides

CORN SALAD *page 105*

Makes 12 servings; Serving size: ½ cup

Calories: 90, Total Fat: 2 gm, Saturated Fat: 0 gm, Monounsaturated Fat: 0 gm, Polyunsaturated Fat: 1 gm, Cholesterol: 0 mg, Protein: 2 gm, Carbohydrate: 17 gm, Dietary Fiber: 1 gm, Sodium: 360 mg

EDAMAME VEGETABLE SALAD *page 106*

Makes 6 servings; Serving size: 1 cup

Calories: 100, Total Fat: 4 gm, Saturated Fat: 0 gm, Monounsaturated Fat: 1 gm, Polyunsaturated Fat: 1 gm, Cholesterol: 0 mg, Protein: 5 gm, Carbohydrate: 10 gm, Dietary Fiber: 5 gm, Sodium: 75 mg

LENTIL & RED PEPPER SALAD *page 108*

Makes 8 servings; Serving size: ½ cup

Calories: 120, Total Fat: 3.5 gm, Saturated Fat: 0.5 gm, Monounsaturated Fat: 2.5 gm, Polyunsaturated Fat: 0 gm, Cholesterol: 0 mg, Protein: 5 gm, Carbohydrate: 16 gm, Dietary Fiber: 5 gm, Sodium: 50 mg

VEGETABLE ORZO *page 109*

Makes 12 servings; Serving size: ½ cup

Calories: 90, Total Fat: 0.5 gm, Saturated Fat: 0 gm, Monounsaturated Fat: 0 gm, Polyunsaturated Fat: 0 gm, Cholesterol: 0 mg, Protein: 4 gm, Carbohydrate: 18 gm, Dietary Fiber: 3 gm, Sodium: 80 mg

THREE BEAN SALSA *page 110*

Makes 12 servings; Serving size: ¾ cup

Calories: 140, Total Fat: 3 gm, Saturated Fat: 0 gm, Monounsaturated Fat: 1.5 gm, Polyunsaturated Fat: 0 gm, Cholesterol: 0 mg, Protein: 7 gm, Carbohydrate: 25 gm, Dietary Fiber: 7 gm, Sodium: 290 mg

MIXED POTATO SALAD *page 112*

Makes 12 servings; Serving size: ½ cup

Calories: 70, Total Fat: 1.5 gm, Saturated Fat: 0 gm, Monounsaturated Fat: 0 gm, Polyunsaturated Fat: 0 gm, Cholesterol: 0 mg, Protein: 2 gm, Carbohydrate: 12 gm, Dietary Fiber: 2 gm, Sodium: 115 mg

CLASSIC MACARONI SALAD *page 113*

Makes 10 servings; Serving size: ½ cup

Calories: 120, Total Fat: 3 gm, Saturated Fat: 0 gm, Monounsaturated Fat: 1 gm, Polyunsaturated Fat: 2 gm, Cholesterol: 0 mg, Protein: 4 gm, Carbohydrate: 20 gm, Dietary Fiber: 2 gm, Sodium: 360 mg

FLAVORFUL COUSCOUS *page 114*

Makes 14 servings; Serving size: ½ cup

Calories: 110, Total Fat: 0 gm, Saturated Fat: 0 gm, Monounsaturated Fat: 0 gm, Polyunsaturated Fat: 0 gm, Cholesterol: 0 mg, Protein: 3 gm, Carbohydrate: 22 gm, Dietary Fiber: 2 gm, Sodium: 130 mg

BOWTIE ZUCCHINI PASTA *page 116*

Makes 25 servings; Serving size: ½ cup

Calories: 90, Total Fat: 1.5 gm, Saturated Fat: 0 gm, Monounsaturated Fat: 0.5 gm, Polyunsaturated Fat: 0 gm, Cholesterol: 0 mg, Protein: 4 gm, Carbohydrate: 15 gm, Dietary Fiber: 2 gm, Sodium: 35 mg

WILD RICE PILAF SALAD *page 117*

Makes 20 servings; Serving size: ½ cup

Calories: 120, Total Fat: 4 gm, Saturated Fat: 0.5 gm, Monounsaturated Fat: 2.5 gm, Polyunsaturated Fat: 0.5 gm, Cholesterol: 0 mg, Protein: 3 gm, Carbohydrate: 18 gm, Dietary Fiber: 2 gm, Sodium: 20 mg

TABOULI SALAD *page 118*

Makes 9 servings; Serving size: ⅔ cup

Calories: 70, Total Fat: 0 gm, Saturated Fat: 0 gm, Monounsaturated Fat: 0 gm, Polyunsaturated Fat: 0 gm, Cholesterol: 0 mg, Protein: 3 gm, Carbohydrate: 15 gm, Dietary Fiber: 4 gm, Sodium: 10 mg

WHEAT BERRY BEAN SALAD *page 120*

Makes 24 servings; Serving size: ½ cup

Calories: 100, Total Fat: 1 gm, Saturated Fat: 0 gm, Monounsaturated Fat: 0 gm, Polyunsaturated Fat: 0 gm, Cholesterol: 0 mg, Protein: 5 gm, Carbohydrate: 20 gm, Dietary Fiber: 5 gm, Sodium: 80 mg

ANGEL HAIR & CABBAGE SALAD *page 121*

Makes 12 servings; Serving size: ½ cup

Calories: 210, Total Fat: 7 gm, Saturated Fat: 1 gm, Monounsaturated Fat: 4.5 gm, Polyunsaturated Fat: 1 gm, Cholesterol: 0 mg, Protein: 6 gm, Carbohydrate: 30 gm, Dietary Fiber: 3 gm, Sodium: 45 mg

GREEK ROTINI SALAD *page 122*

Makes 12 servings; Serving size: 1 cup

Calories: 160, Total Fat: 3 gm, Saturated Fat: 1 gm, Monounsaturated Fat: 1 gm, Polyunsaturated Fat: 0 gm, Cholesterol: 5 mg, Protein: 9 gm, Carbohydrate: 30 gm, Dietary Fiber: 5 gm, Sodium: 105 mg

Kugels & Latkes

SWEET NOODLE KUGEL *page 127*

Makes 16 servings; Serving size: 1 piece

Calories: 70, Total Fat: 1 gm, Saturated Fat: 0 gm, Monounsaturated Fat: 0 gm, Polyunsaturated Fat: 0 gm, Cholesterol: 20 mg, Protein: 2 gm, Carbohydrate: 14 gm, Dietary Fiber: <1 gm, Sodium: 15 mg

SALT & PEPPER NOODLE KUGEL *page 128*

Makes 16 servings; Serving size: 1 piece

Calories: 110, Total Fat: 3 gm, Saturated Fat: 0.5 gm, Monounsaturated Fat: 1.5 gm, Polyunsaturated Fat: 0.5 gm, Cholesterol: 30 mg, Protein: 4 gm, Carbohydrate: 15 gm, Dietary Fiber: <1 gm, Sodium: 170 mg

CARROT & PARSNIP LATKES *page 130*

Makes 12 servings; Serving size: 2 latkes

Calories: 45, Total Fat: 1 gm, Saturated Fat: 0 gm, Monounsaturated Fat: 0 gm, Polyunsaturated Fat: 0 gm, Cholesterol: 15 mg, Protein: 2 gm, Carbohydrate: 8 gm, Dietary Fiber: 1 gm, Sodium: 130 mg

VEGETABLE KUGEL *page 131*

Makes 20 servings; Serving size: 1 piece

Calories: 35, Total Fat: 1 gm, Saturated Fat: 0 gm, Monounsaturated Fat: 0.5 gm, Polyunsaturated Fat: 0 gm, Cholesterol: 10 mg, Protein: 2 gm, Carbohydrate: 5 gm, Dietary Fiber: 1 gm, Sodium: 115 mg

POTATO LATKES page 132

Makes 8 servings; Serving size: 2 latkes

Calories: 70, Total Fat: 0.5 gm, Saturated Fat: 0 gm, Monounsaturated Fat: 0 gm, Polyunsaturated Fat: 0 gm, Cholesterol: 0 mg, Protein: 3 gm, Carbohydrate: 14 gm, Dietary Fiber: 2 gm, Sodium: 160 mg

SWEET POTATO & APPLE LATKES page 134

Makes 12 servings; Serving size: 2 latkes

Calories: 60, Total Fat: 0 gm, Saturated Fat: 0 gm, Monounsaturated Fat: 0 gm, Polyunsaturated Fat: 0 gm, Cholesterol: 0 gm, Protein: 2 gm, Carbohydrate: 13 gm, Dietary Fiber: 1 gm, Sodium: 20 mg

CRISP POTATO KUGEL page 135

Makes 20 servings; Serving size: 1 piece

Calories: 70, Total Fat: 1.5 gm, Saturated Fat: 0 gm, Monounsaturated Fat: 1 gm, Polyunsaturated Fat: 0 gm, Cholesterol: 0 mg, Protein: 2 gm, Carbohydrate: 11 gm, Dietary Fiber: 1 gm, Sodium: 190 mg

CARROT KUGEL page 136

Makes 9 servings; Serving size: 1 piece

Calories: 100, Total Fat: 1.5 gm, Saturated Fat: 0 gm, Monounsaturated Fat: 0 gm, Polyunsaturated Fat: 0 gm, Cholesterol: 20 mg, Protein: 3 gm, Carbohydrate: 18 gm, Dietary Fiber: 2 gm, Sodium: 330 mg

SPINACH NOODLE KUGEL page 138

Makes 16 servings; Serving size: 1 piece

Calories: 100, Total Fat: 2 gm, Saturated Fat: 0 gm, Monounsaturated Fat: 0 gm, Polyunsaturated Fat: 0.5 gm, Cholesterol: 30 mg, Protein: 5 gm, Carbohydrate: 16 gm, Dietary Fiber: 1 gm, Sodium: 120 mg

PINEAPPLE KUGEL page 139

Makes 9 servings; Serving size: 1 piece

Calories: 135, Total Fat: 1 gm, Saturated Fat: 0 gm, Monounsaturated Fat: 0 gm, Polyunsaturated Fat: 0 gm, Cholesterol: 40 mg, Protein: 4 gm, Carbohydrate: 28 gm, Dietary Fiber: <1 gm, Sodium: 60 mg

Appendix

Poultry & Meat

CRISPY BAKED CHICKEN *page 145*
Makes 6 servings; Serving size: 1 chicken breast
Calories: 190, Total Fat: 3.5 gm, Saturated Fat: 1 gm, Monounsaturated Fat: 1 gm, Polyunsaturated Fat: 0.5 gm, Cholesterol: 75 mg, Protein: 26 gm, Carbohydrate: 13 gm, Dietary Fiber: <1 gm, Sodium: 350 mg

VERSATILE CHICKEN BREAST *page 146*
Makes 4 servings; Serving size: 1 chicken breast
Calories: 130, Total Fat: 3 gm, Saturated Fat: 0.5 gm, Monounsaturated Fat: 1 gm, Polyunsaturated Fat: 0 gm, Cholesterol: 75 mg, Protein: 24 gm, Carbohydrate: 0 gm, Dietary Fiber: 0 gm, Sodium: 420 mg

ASIAN CHICKEN TOPPER *page 147*
Makes 6 servings; Serving size: ¼ cup
Calories: 50, Total Fat: 2.5 gm, Saturated Fat: 0 gm, Monounsaturated Fat: 1.5 gm, Polyunsaturated Fat: 0.5 gm, Cholesterol: 0 mg, Protein: 3 gm, Carbohydrate: 5 gm, Dietary Fiber: 3 gm, Sodium: 60 mg

CABBAGE-APPLE CHICKEN TOPPER *page 148*
Makes 6 servings; Serving size: ¼ cup
Calories: 35, Total Fat: 1 gm, Saturated Fat: 0 gm, Monounsaturated Fat: 0.5 gm, Polyunsaturated Fat: 0 gm, Cholesterol: 0 mg, Protein: <1 gm, Carbohydrate: 7 gm, Dietary Fiber: 2 gm, Sodium: 10 mg

COLORED PEPPER CHICKEN TOPPER *page 148*
Makes 6 servings; Serving size: ¼ cup
Calories: 40, Total Fat: 2.5 gm, Saturated Fat: 0 gm, Monounsaturated Fat: 1.5 gm, Polyunsaturated Fat: 0 gm, Cholesterol: 0 mg, Protein: <1 gm, Carbohydrate: 4 gm, Dietary Fiber: 1 gm, Sodium: 0 mg

CHICKEN SCALLOPINE WITH MARSALA *page 149*

Makes 5 servings; Serving size: 3 ounces

Calories: 180, Total Fat: 8 gm, Saturated Fat: 1 gm, Monounsaturated Fat: 4.5 gm, Polyunsaturated Fat: 1 gm, Cholesterol: 60 mg, Protein: 20 gm, Carbohydrate: 6 gm, Dietary Fiber: 0 gm, Sodium: 180 mg

ITALIAN TURKEY SAUTÉ *page 150*

Makes 4 servings; Serving size: 1 cup

Calories: 220, Total Fat: 5 gm, Saturated Fat: 1 gm, Monounsaturated Fat: 2.5 gm, Polyunsaturated Fat: 1 gm, Cholesterol: 95 mg, Protein: 34 gm, Carbohydrate: 9 gm, Dietary Fiber: 2 gm, Sodium: 250 mg

HAWAIIAN TURKEY SALAD *page 152*

Makes 8 servings; Serving size: 1 cup

Calories: 100, Total Fat: 2.5 gm, Saturated Fat: 0 gm, Monounsaturated Fat: 0 gm, Polyunsaturated Fat: 1 gm, Cholesterol: 35 mg, Protein: 13 gm, Carbohydrate: 9 gm, Dietary Fiber: 1 gm, Sodium: 130 mg

KALE-STUFFED CHICKEN ROLL *page 153*

Makes 4 servings; Serving size: 1 chicken breast

Calories: 310, Total Fat: 10 gm, Saturated Fat: 1.5 gm, Monounsaturated Fat: 4 gm, Polyunsaturated Fat: 2.5 gm, Cholesterol: 85 mg, Protein: 32 gm, Carbohydrate: 25 gm, Dietary Fiber: 5 gm, Sodium: 390 mg

BALSAMIC LEMON CHICKEN *page 154*

Makes 6 servings; Serving size: 1 chicken breast

Calories: 150, Total Fat: 3 gm, Saturated Fat: 0.5 gm, Monounsaturated Fat: 1 gm, Polyunsaturated Fat: 0 gm, Cholesterol: 75 mg, Protein: 25 gm, Carbohydrate: 6 gm, Dietary Fiber: 1 gm, Sodium: 135 mg

ROSEMARY CHICKEN & WHITE BEAN STEW *page 156*

Makes 5 servings; Serving size: 1 ½ cups

Calories: 260, Total Fat: 6 gm, Saturated Fat: 1 gm, Monounsaturated Fat: 2.5 gm, Polyunsaturated Fat: 1 gm, Cholesterol: 60 gm, Protein: 27 gm, Carbohydrate: 26 gm, Dietary Fiber: 9 gm, Sodium: 760 mg

Appendix

BEEF & ASPARAGUS STIR-FRY *page 157*

Makes 6 servings; Serving size: 1 cup

Calories: 190, Total Fat: 8 gm, Saturated Fat: 3 gm, Monounsaturated Fat: 3.5 gm, Polyunsaturated Fat: 0 gm, Cholesterol: 65 mg, Protein: 23 gm, Carbohydrate: 5 gm, Dietary Fiber: 1 gm, Sodium: 85 mg

BRIGHT LEMON CHICKEN *page 158*

Makes 4 servings; Serving size: 1 chicken breast

Calories: 290, Total Fat: 8 gm, Saturated Fat: 1.5 gm, Monounsaturated Fat: 3.5 gm, Polyunsaturated Fat: 1 gm, Cholesterol: 90 mg, Protein: 34 gm, Carbohydrate: 20 gm, Dietary Fiber: <1 gm, Sodium: 260 mg

TURKEY & APPLE WRAP *page 160*

Makes 4 servings; Serving size: 1 wrap

Calories: 290, Total Fat: 7 gm, Saturated Fat: 3 gm, Monounsaturated Fat: 2 gm, Polyunsaturated Fat: 1.5 gm, Cholesterol: 60 mg, Protein: 30 gm, Carbohydrate: 28 gm, Dietary Fiber: 6 gm, Sodium: 370 mg

TURKEY & MIXED BEAN CHILI *page 161*

Makes 8 servings; Serving size: 1 cup

Calories: 180, Total Fat: 3 gm, Saturated Fat: 0.5 gm, Monounsaturated Fat: 1.5 gm, Polyunsaturated Fat: 0.5 gm, Cholesterol: 27 gm, Protein: 19 gm, Carbohydrate: 29 gm, Dietary Fiber: 9 gm, Sodium: 380 mg

ORANGE GRILLED CHICKEN SALAD *page 162*

Makes 6 servings; Serving size: 1 cup

Calories: 230, Total Fat: 11 gm, Saturated Fat: 1.5 gm, Monounsaturated Fat: 7 gm, Polyunsaturated Fat: 1.5 gm, Cholesterol: 50 mg, Protein: 17 gm, Carbohydrate: 13 gm, Dietary Fiber: 2 gm, Sodium: 100 mg

HOME-STYLE CHICKEN PACKETS *page 164*

Makes 4 servings; Serving size: 1 chicken breast

Calories: 170, Total Fat: 3.5 gm, Saturated Fat: 0.5 gm, Monounsaturated Fat: 1 gm, Polyunsaturated Fat: 0.5 gm, Cholesterol: 75 mg, Protein: 27 gm, Carbohydrate: 8 gm, Dietary Fiber: 3 gm, Sodium: 230 mg

MEDITERRANEAN CHICKEN & RICE CASSEROLE *page 165*

Makes 6 servings; Serving size: 3 chicken strips with ½ cup rice mixture

Calories: 300, Total Fat: 6 gm, Saturated Fat: 1 gm, Monounsaturated Fat: 3 gm, Polyunsaturated Fat: 1 gm, Cholesterol: 75 mg, Protein: 29 gm, Carbohydrate: 32 gm, Dietary Fiber: 3 gm, Sodium: 270 mg

POMEGRANATE-ORANGE GLAZED TURKEY *page 166*

Makes 16 servings; Serving size: 3 ounces

Calories: 130, Total Fat: 2 gm, Saturated Fat: 0 gm, Monounsaturated Fat: 0 gm, Polyunsaturated Fat: 0 gm, Cholesterol: 55 mg, Protein: 23 gm, Carbohydrate: 5 gm, Dietary Fiber: 0 gm, Sodium: 75 mg

SWEET CURRIED CHICKEN *page 168*

Makes 8 servings; Serving size: 1 chicken quarter

Calories: 300, Total Fat: 10 gm, Saturated Fat: 2 gm, Monounsaturated Fat: 2.5 gm, Polyunsaturated Fat: 2.5 gm, Cholesterol: 175 mg, Protein: 47 gm, Carbohydrate: 10 gm, Dietary Fiber: <1 gm, Sodium: 270 mg

CHERRY & APRICOT TURKEY CASSEROLE *page 169*

Makes 6 servings; Serving size: 1 cup

Calories: 340, Total Fat: 5 gm, Saturated Fat: 1 gm, Monounsaturated Fat: 2 gm, Polyunsaturated Fat: 2 gm, Cholesterol: 65 mg, Protein: 32 gm, Carbohydrate: 40 gm, Dietary Fiber: 3 gm, Sodium: 230 mg

CHICKEN & BROCCOLI STIR-FRY *page 170*

Makes 4 servings; Serving size: 1 cup

Calories: 170, Total Fat: 5 gm, Saturated Fat: 1 gm, Monounsaturated Fat: 2 gm, Polyunsaturated Fat: 0.5 gm, Cholesterol: 55 mg, Protein: 21 gm, Carbohydrate: 10 gm, Dietary Fiber: 2 gm, Sodium: 370 mg

MARINATED BEEF KEBOBS *page 172*

Makes 2 servings; Serving size: 2 kebobs

Calories: 360, Total Fat: 21 gm, Saturated Fat: 4 gm, Monounsaturated Fat: 13 gm, Polyunsaturated Fat: 2 gm, Cholesterol: 55 mg, Protein: 22 gm, Carbohydrate: 23 gm, Dietary Fiber: 5 gm, Sodium: 85 mg

Appendix

TASTY CHICKEN SLIDERS *page 173*

Makes 10 servings; Serving size: 2 sliders

Calories: 90, Total Fat: 3.5 gm, Saturated Fat: 1 gm, Monounsaturated Fat: 1.5 gm, Polyunsaturated Fat: 0.5 gm, Cholesterol: 40 mg, Protein: 9 gm, Carbohydrate: 4 gm, Dietary Fiber: <1 gm, Sodium: 40 mg

BEEF GOULASH *page 174*

Makes 8 servings; Serving size: 1 cup

Calories: 260, Total Fat: 12 gm, Saturated Fat: 5 gm, Monounsaturated Fat: 6 gm, Polyunsaturated Fat: 1 gm, Cholesterol: 100 mg, Protein: 30 gm, Carbohydrate: 9 gm, Dietary Fiber: 2 gm, Sodium: 192 mg

CHICKEN POT PIE *page 176*

Makes 6 servings; Serving size: 1 piece

Calories: 260, Total Fat: 17 gm, Saturated Fat: 2.5 gm, Monounsaturated Fat: 11 gm, Polyunsaturated Fat: 2 gm, Cholesterol: 20 mg, Protein: 11 gm, Carbohydrate: 17 gm, Dietary Fiber: 2 gm, Sodium: 240 mg

CHICKEN PAPRIKASH *page 178*

Makes 8 servings; Serving size: 1 chicken breast

Calories: 330, Total Fat: 8 gm, Saturated Fat: 1.5 gm, Monounsaturated Fat: 3 gm, Polyunsaturated Fat: 1.5 gm, Cholesterol: 150 mg, Protein: 52 gm, Carbohydrate: 9 gm, Dietary Fiber: 3 gm, Sodium: 300 mg

Fish

ZESTY SALMON FILLETS *page 183*

Makes 4 servings; Serving size: 1 fillet

Calories: 100, Total Fat: 5 gm, Saturated Fat: 1 gm, Monounsaturated Fat: 1.5 gm, Polyunsaturated Fat: 2 gm, Cholesterol: 30 mg, Protein: 12 gm, Carbohydrate: 2 gm, Dietary Fiber: 0 gm, Sodium: 170 mg

MAHI-MAHI TACOS WITH TROPICAL SALSA *page 184*

Makes 4 servings; Serving size: 2 tacos

Calories: 210, Total Fat: 2 gm, Saturated Fat: 0 gm, Monounsaturated Fat: 0 gm, Polyunsaturated Fat: 0 gm, Cholesterol: 85 mg, Protein: 23 gm, Carbohydrate: 24 gm, Dietary Fiber: 3 gm, Sodium: 120 mg

GRILLED SALMON WITH HONEY MUSTARD DILL SAUCE *page 186*

Makes 4 servings; Serving size: 1 salmon steak

Calories: 270, Total Fat: 11 gm, Saturated Fat: 1.5 gm, Monounsaturated Fat: 3.5 gm, Polyunsaturated Fat: 4.5 gm, Cholesterol: 95 mg, Protein: 36 gm, Carbohydrate: 4 gm, Dietary Fiber: 0 gm, Sodium: 430 mg

TUNA NOODLE CASSEROLE *page 187*

Makes 4 servings; Serving size: 1 cup

Calories: 300, Total Fat: 9 gm, Saturated Fat: 4.5 gm, Monounsaturated Fat: 2.5 gm, Polyunsaturated Fat: 1 gm, Cholesterol: 60 mg, Protein: 21 gm, Carbohydrate: 34 gm, Dietary Fiber: 2 gm, Sodium: 440 mg

BRUSCHETTA BAKED TILAPIA *page 188*

Makes 4 servings; Serving size: 1 fillets

Calories: 130, Total Fat: 3 gm, Saturated Fat: 1 gm, Monounsaturated Fat: 1.5 gm, Polyunsaturated Fat: 0.5 gm, Cholesterol: 55 mg, Protein: 23 gm, Carbohydrate: 3 gm, Dietary Fiber: <1 gm, Sodium: 170 mg

MEDITERRANEAN TUNA POUCHES *page 190*

Makes 6 servings; Serving size: 1 tuna pouch

Calories: 200, Total Fat: 4 gm, Saturated Fat: 1 gm, Monounsaturated Fat: 1 gm, Polyunsaturated Fat: 1 gm, Cholesterol: 30 mg, Protein: 20 gm, Carbohydrate: 23 gm, Dietary Fiber: 4 gm, Sodium: 440 mg

MOROCCAN SALMON *page 191*

Makes 8 servings; Serving size: 1 fillet

Calories: 240, Total Fat: 14 gm, Saturated Fat: 2 gm, Monounsaturated Fat: 7 gm, Polyunsaturated Fat: 3.5 gm, Cholesterol: 65 mg, Protein: 23 gm, Carbohydrate: 5 gm, Dietary Fiber: 1 gm, Sodium: 90 mg

Appendix

LEMON GARLIC SALMON *page 192*

Makes 2 servings; Serving size: 1 fillet

Calories: 300, Total Fat: 18 gm, Saturated Fat: 2.5 gm, Monounsaturated Fat: 9 gm, Polyunsaturated Fat: 5 gm, Cholesterol: 95 mg, Protein: 34 gm, Carbohydrate: <1 gm, Dietary Fiber: 0 gm, Sodium: 75 mg

BROILED TILAPIA WITH ZESTY MANDARIN ORANGE RELISH *page 194*

Makes 4 servings; Serving size: 1 fillet

Calories: 150, Total Fat: 2 gm, Saturated Fat: 0.5 gm, Monounsaturated Fat: 0.5 gm, Polyunsaturated Fat: 0 gm, Cholesterol: 55 mg, Protein: 24 gm, Carbohydrate: 9 gm, Dietary Fiber: 1 gm, Sodium: 65 mg

LEMON PEPPER HALIBUT WITH LINGUINE *page 195*

Makes 4 servings; Serving size: 1 fillet over linguine

Calories: 290, Total Fat: 6 gm, Saturated Fat: 1 gm, Monounsaturated Fat: 1.5 gm, Polyunsaturated Fat: 2.5 gm, Cholesterol: 40 mg, Protein: 31 gm, Carbohydrate: 28 gm, Dietary Fiber: 4 gm, Sodium: 220 mg

BROILED FISH FILLETS WITH MUSTARD *page 196*

Makes 4 servings; Serving size: 1 fillet

Calories: 120, Total Fat: 2.5 gm, Saturated Fat: 0.5 gm, Monounsaturated Fat: 0 gm, Polyunsaturated Fat: 1 gm, Cholesterol: 70 mg, Protein: 24 gm, Carbohydrate: 3 gm, Dietary Fiber: 1 gm, Sodium: 230 mg

ORANGE-GLAZED SALMON *page 198*

Makes 4 servings; Serving size: 1 fillet

Calories: 210, Total Fat: 10 gm, Saturated Fat: 1.5 gm, Monounsaturated Fat: 3.5 gm, Polyunsaturated Fat: 4 gm, Cholesterol: 65 mg, Protein: 23 gm, Carbohydrate: 6 gm, Dietary Fiber: 0 gm, Sodium: 350 mg

OPEN-FACED TUNA MELT *page 199*

Makes 4 servings; Serving size: 1 open-faced slice

Calories: 300, Total Fat: 13 gm, Saturated Fat: 5 gm, Monounsaturated Fat: 1.5 gm, Polyunsaturated Fat: 3.5 gm, Cholesterol: 60 mg, Protein: 31 gm, Carbohydrate: 17 gm, Dietary Fiber: 2 gm, Sodium: 810 mg

VEGETABLE & FISH STIR-FRY *page 200*

Makes 6 servings; Serving size: 1 cup

Calories: 170, Total Fat: 6 gm, Saturated Fat: 1 gm, Monounsaturated Fat: 3 gm, Polyunsaturated Fat: 1 gm, Cholesterol: 60 mg, Protein: 16 gm, Carbohydrate: 14 gm, Dietary Fiber: 2 gm, Sodium: 110 mg

TUNA BOATS *page 201*

Makes 4 servings; Serving size: 1 boat

Calories: 80, Total Fat: 2 gm, Saturated Fat: 0.5 gm, Monounsaturated Fat: 0.5 gm, Polyunsaturated Fat: 1 gm, Cholesterol: 15 mg, Protein: 12 gm, Carbohydrate: 4 gm, Dietary Fiber: 1 gm, Sodium: 170 mg

Dairy & Pasta Entrees

SPINACH PARMESAN LASAGNA *page 207*

Makes 4 servings; Serving size: 2 lasagna rolls

Calories: 320, Total Fat: 3.5 gm, Saturated Fat: 0 gm, Monounsaturated Fat: 1 gm, Polyunsaturated Fat: 1 gm, Cholesterol: <5 mg, Protein: 21 gm, Carbohydrate: 50 gm, Dietary Fiber: 5 gm, Sodium: 730 mg

SHAKSHUKA *page 208*

Makes 6 servings; Serving size: 1 cup

Calories: 140, Total Fat: 7 gm, Saturated Fat: 2 gm, Monounsaturated Fat: 3.5 gm, Polyunsaturated Fat: 1 gm, Cholesterol: 185 mg, Protein: 8 gm, Carbohydrate: 10 gm, Dietary Fiber: 3 gm, Sodium: 210 mg

VEGETABLE STRATA *page 210*

Makes 6 servings; Serving size: 1 piece

Calories: 110, Total Fat: 5 gm, Saturated Fat: 1.5 gm, Monounsaturated Fat: 2 gm, Polyunsaturated Fat: 1 gm, Cholesterol: 125 mg, Protein: 8 gm, Carbohydrate: 8 gm, Dietary Fiber: 1 gm, Sodium: 120 mg

BROCCOLI QUICHE *page 211*

Makes 8 servings; Serving size: 1 slice

Calories: 80, Total Fat: 3 gm, Saturated Fat: 1 gm, Monounsaturated Fat: 0 gm, Polyunsaturated Fat: 0 gm, Cholesterol: 30 mg, Protein: 9 gm, Carbohydrate: 5 gm, Dietary Fiber: <1 gm, Sodium: 300 mg

Appendix

PITA PIZZA page 212

Makes 6 servings; Serving size: 1 pita pizza

Calories: 280, Total Fat: 7 gm, Saturated Fat: 4 gm, Monounsaturated Fat: 1 gm, Polyunsaturated Fat: 1 gm, Cholesterol: 25 mg, Protein: 14 gm, Carbohydrate: 44 gm, Dietary Fiber: 5 gm, Sodium: 650 mg

CHEESY ARTICHOKE & TOMATO FRITTATA page 214

Makes 8 servings; Serving size: 1 slice

Calories: 100, Total Fat: 4 gm, Saturated Fat: 2 gm, Monounsaturated Fat: 1 gm, Polyunsaturated Fat: 0.5 gm, Cholesterol: 75 mg, Protein: 8 gm, Carbohydrate: 8 gm, Dietary Fiber: 3 gm, Sodium: 220 mg

TOMATO ZUCCHINI PARMESAN page 215

Makes 6 servings; Serving size: 1 cup

Calories: 180, Total Fat: 8 gm, Saturated Fat: 3 gm, Monounsaturated Fat: 1 gm, Polyunsaturated Fat: 0 gm, Cholesterol: 45 mg, Protein: 15 gm, Carbohydrate: 9 gm, Dietary Fiber: 2 gm, Sodium: 610 mg

EGGPLANT CASSEROLE page 216

Makes 6 servings; Serving size: 1 cup

Calories: 320, Total Fat: 12 gm, Saturated Fat: 3.5 gm, Monounsaturated Fat: 3.5 gm, Polyunsaturated Fat: 1 gm, Cholesterol: 15 mg, Protein: 18 gm, Carbohydrate: 37 gm, Dietary Fiber: 8 gm, Sodium: 650 mg

FETTUCCINI WITH VEGETABLES page 218

Makes 5 servings; Serving size: 1 cup

Calories: 170, Total Fat: 3.5 gm, Saturated Fat: 1 gm, Monounsaturated Fat: 1 gm, Polyunsaturated Fat: 0 gm, Cholesterol: 28 mg, Protein: 8 gm, Carbohydrate: 27 gm, Dietary Fiber: 4 gm, Sodium: 170 mg

Vegetarian

TOFU-STUFFED MANICOTTI SHELLS *page 223*
Makes 12 servings; Serving size: 2 stuffed shells
Calories: 180, Total Fat: 6 gm, Saturated Fat: 2 gm, Monounsaturated Fat: 0 gm, Polyunsaturated Fat: 0.5 gm, Cholesterol: 10 mg, Protein: 13 gm, Carbohydrate: 21 gm, Dietary Fiber: 2 gm, Sodium: 430 mg

ORZO-STUFFED PEPPERS *page 224*
Makes 6 servings; Serving size: 1 stuffed pepper
Calories: 280, Total Fat: 7 gm, Saturated Fat: 3 gm, Monounsaturated Fat: 2 gm, Polyunsaturated Fat: 0.5 gm, Cholesterol: 15 mg, Protein: 13 gm, Carbohydrate: 42 gm, Dietary Fiber: 4 gm, Sodium: 280 mg

TEMPEH FAJITAS *page 226*
Makes 12 servings; Serving size: 1 fajita
Calories: 220, Total Fat: 9 gm, Saturated Fat: 3 gm, Monounsaturated Fat: 3 gm, Polyunsaturated Fat: 2 gm, Cholesterol: 0 mg, Protein: 12 gm, Carbohydrate: 25 gm, Dietary Fiber: 5 gm, Sodium: 280 mg

VEGETABLE CUTLETS *page 227*
Makes 8 servings; Serving size: 2 cutlets
Calories: 130, Total Fat: 1.5 gm, Saturated Fat: 0 gm, Monounsaturated Fat: 0 gm, Polyunsaturated Fat: 0.5 gm, Cholesterol: 25 mg, Protein: 7 gm, Carbohydrate: 24 gm, Dietary Fiber: 4 gm, Sodium: 200 mg

TOFU VEGGIE BURGERS *page 228*
Makes 16 servings; Serving size: 1 burger
Calories: 110, Total Fat: 4 gm, Saturated Fat: 0.5 gm, Monounsaturated Fat: 2 gm, Polyunsaturated Fat: 1 gm, Cholesterol: 0 mg, Protein: 5 gm, Carbohydrate: 15 gm, Dietary Fiber: 2 gm, Sodium: 110 mg

LENTIL-STUFFED TOMATOES *page 230*

Makes 4 servings; Serving size: 1 stuffed tomato
Calories: 100, Total Fat: 1 gm, Saturated Fat: 0 gm, Monounsaturated Fat: 0 gm,
Polyunsaturated Fat: 0 gm, Cholesterol: 0 gm, Protein: 6 gm, Carbohydrate: 18 gm, Dietary Fiber: 4 gm,
Sodium: 330 mg

SPICY BEAN BURGERS *page 231*

Makes 4 servings; Serving size: 1 burger
Calories: 230, Total Fat: 6 gm, Saturated Fat: 2 gm, Monounsaturated Fat: 3 gm,
Polyunsaturated Fat: 0 gm, Cholesterol: 10 mg, Protein: 13 gm, Carbohydrate: 29 gm, Dietary Fiber: 8 gm,
Sodium: 230 mg

TOFU CRISP OVER NOODLES *page 232*

Makes 4 servings; Serving size: 1 tofu crisp with 1 cup noodles
Calories: 350, Total Fat: 10 gm, Saturated Fat: 1.5 gm, Monounsaturated Fat: 5 gm,
Polyunsaturated Fat: 1.5 gm, Cholesterol: 0 mg, Protein: 20 gm, Carbohydrate: 50 gm, Dietary Fiber: 6 gm,
Sodium: 140 mg

MEDITERRANEAN VEGGIE BURGERS *page 234*

Makes 4 servings; Serving size: 1 burger
Calories: 310, Total Fat: 7.5 gm, Saturated Fat: 1 gm, Monounsaturated Fat: 3.5 gm,
Polyunsaturated Fat: 1 gm, Cholesterol: 0 mg, Protein: 12 gm, Carbohydrate: 52 gm, Dietary Fiber: 9 gm,
Sodium: 760 mg

TOFU CHILI *page 235*

Makes 8 servings; Serving size: 1 cup
Calories: 180, Total Fat: 3 gm, Saturated Fat: 0.5 gm, Monounsaturated Fat: 1 gm,
Polyunsaturated Fat: 1.5 gm, Cholesterol: 0 mg, Protein: 13 gm, Carbohydrate: 29 gm, Dietary Fiber: 9 gm,
Sodium: 450 mg

Breakfast

CHEESY EGG QUESADILLAS *page 241*

Makes 4 servings; Serving size: 1 quesadilla

Calories: 190, Total Fat: 5 gm, Saturated Fat: 2 gm, Monounsaturated Fat: 1 gm, Polyunsaturated Fat: 0.5 gm, Cholesterol: 100 mg, Protein: 13 gm, Carbohydrate: 24 gm, Dietary Fiber: 4 gm, Sodium: 270 mg

VEGETABLE TOFU SCRAMBLE *page 242*

Makes 3 servings; Serving size: 1 cup

Calories: 80, Total Fat: 2 gm, Saturated Fat: 0 gm, Monounsaturated Fat: 0.5 gm, Polyunsaturated Fat: 0.5 gm, Cholesterol: 0 mg, Protein: 9 gm, Carbohydrate: 6 gm, Dietary Fiber: 1 gm, Sodium: 640 mg

VEGGIE EGG DELIGHT *page 244*

Makes 6 servings; Serving size: 1 cup

Calories: 110, Total Fat: 6 gm, Saturated Fat: 1.5 gm, Monounsaturated Fat: 3 gm, Polyunsaturated Fat: 1 gm, Cholesterol: 95 mg, Protein: 8 gm, Carbohydrate: 8 gm, Dietary Fiber: 2 gm, Sodium: 200 mg

BANANA NUT PANCAKES *page 245*

Makes 10 servings; Serving size: 2 pancakes

Calories: 160, Total Fat: 6 gm, Saturated Fat: 1 gm, Monounsaturated Fat: 1.5 gm, Polyunsaturated Fat: 3 gm, Cholesterol: 0 mg, Protein: 5 gm, Carbohydrate: 24 gm, Dietary Fiber: 3 gm, Sodium: 210 mg

WHOLE WHEAT CHOCOLATE PANCAKES *page 246*

Makes 10 servings; Serving size: 2 pancakes

Calories: 140, Total Fat: 4 gm, Saturated Fat: 2 gm, Monounsaturated Fat: 1 gm, Polyunsaturated Fat: 1 gm, Cholesterol: 0 mg, Protein: 6 gm, Carbohydrate: 23 gm, Dietary Fiber: 4 gm, Sodium: 220 mg

Appendix

FRUIT FRENCH TOAST CASSEROLE *page 248*

Makes 6 servings; Serving size: 1 piece
Calories: 160, Total Fat: 3 gm, Saturated Fat: 1 gm, Monounsaturated Fat: 1 gm,
Polyunsaturated Fat: 1 gm, Cholesterol: 65 mg, Protein: 9 gm, Carbohydrate: 25 gm, Dietary Fiber: 2 gm,
Sodium: 180 mg

Muffins & Breads

APPLE CRAISIN MUFFINS *page 253*

Makes 12 servings; Serving size: 1 muffin
Calories: 100, Total Fat: 0.5 gm, Saturated Fat: 0 gm, Monounsaturated Fat: 0 gm,
Polyunsaturated Fat: 0 gm, Cholesterol: 0 mg, Protein: 4 gm, Carbohydrate: 20 gm, Dietary Fiber: 3 gm,
Sodium: 250 mg

CINNAMON RAISIN BREAD *page 254*

Makes 20 servings; Serving size: 1 slice
Calories: 90, Total Fat: 0 gm, Saturated Fat: 0 gm, Monounsaturated Fat: 0 gm, Polyunsaturated Fat: 0 gm,
Cholesterol: 0 mg, Protein: 2 gm, Carbohydrate: 20 gm, Dietary Fiber: 1 gm, Sodium: 140 mg

CORN MUFFINS *page 256*

Makes 12 servings; Serving size: 1 muffin
Calories: 100, Total Fat: 1 gm, Saturated Fat: 0 gm, Monounsaturated Fat: 0 gm,
Polyunsaturated Fat: 0 gm, Cholesterol: 15 mg, Protein: 3 gm, Carbohydrate: 21 gm, Dietary Fiber: 2 gm,
Sodium: 240 mg

BANANA OATMEAL MUFFINS *page 257*

Makes 12 servings; Serving size: 1 muffin
Calories: 170, Total Fat: 4 gm, Saturated Fat: 0 gm, Monounsaturated Fat: 0.5 gm,
Polyunsaturated Fat: 2.5 gm, Cholesterol: 0 mg, Protein: 4 gm, Carbohydrate: 32 gm, Dietary Fiber: 3 gm,
Sodium: 250 mg

PUMPKIN MUFFINS *page 258*

Makes 12 servings; Serving size: 1 muffin
Calories: 130, Total Fat: 3.5 gm, Saturated Fat: 0 gm, Monounsaturated Fat: 0 gm,
Polyunsaturated Fat: 2.5 gm, Cholesterol: 0 mg, Protein: 3 gm, Carbohydrate: 24 gm, Dietary Fiber: 3 gm,
Sodium: 270 mg

CARROT RAISIN MUFFINS *page 260*

Makes 12 servings; Serving size: 1 muffin

Calories: 120, Total Fat: 0.5 gm, Saturated Fat: 0 gm, Monounsaturated Fat: 0 gm, Polyunsaturated Fat: 0 gm, Cholesterol: 0 mg, Protein: 4 gm, Carbohydrate: 26 gm, Dietary Fiber: 3 gm, Sodium: 75 mg

PEANUT BUTTER BRAN MUFFINS *page 261*

Makes 12 servings; Serving size: 1 muffin

Calories: 130, Total Fat: 4 gm, Saturated Fat: 1 gm, Monounsaturated Fat: 1.5 gm, Polyunsaturated Fat: 1 gm, Cholesterol: 15 mg, Protein: 6 gm, Carbohydrate: 21 gm, Dietary Fiber: 3 gm, Sodium: 120 mg

ZUCCHINI CARROT BREAD *page 262*

Makes 20 servings; Serving size: 1 slice

Calories: 100, Total Fat: 0 gm, Saturated Fat: 0 gm, Monounsaturated Fat: 0 gm, Polyunsaturated Fat: 0 gm, Cholesterol: 0 mg, Protein: 3 gm, Carbohydrate: 21 gm, Dietary Fiber: 2 gm, Sodium: 210 mg

BLUEBERRY OAT BRAN MUFFIN *page 264*

Makes 12 servings; Serving size: 1 muffin

Calories: 70, Total Fat: 1 gm, Saturated Fat: 0 gm, Monounsaturated Fat: 0 gm, Polyunsaturated Fat: 0 gm, Cholesterol: 0 mg, Protein: 3 gm, Carbohydrate: 15 gm, Dietary Fiber: 2 gm, Sodium: 80 mg

WALNUT DATE BREAD *page 265*

Makes 14 servings; Serving size: 1 slice

Calories: 125, Total Fat: 3 gm, Saturated Fat: 0 gm, Monounsaturated Fat: 0 gm, Polyunsaturated Fat: 2 gm, Cholesterol: 0 mg, Protein: 4 gm, Carbohydrate: 22 gm, Dietary Fiber: 3 gm, Sodium: 210 mg

Desserts

COCOA PEANUT BUTTER CRUNCH BALLS *page 271*

Makes 25 servings; Serving size: 2 crunch balls

Calories: 130, Total Fat: 5 gm, Saturated Fat: 1 gm, Monounsaturated Fat: 0 gm, Polyunsaturated Fat: 0 gm, Cholesterol: 0 mg, Protein: 4 gm, Carbohydrate: 19 gm, Dietary Fiber: 3 gm, Sodium: 200 mg

Appendix

QUICK & EASY BROWN SUGAR COOKIES *page 272*

Makes 14 servings; Serving size: 2 cookies

Calories: 130, Total Fat: 6 gm, Saturated Fat: 1 gm, Monounsaturated Fat: 3.5 gm, Polyunsaturated Fat: 2 gm, Cholesterol: 0 mg, Protein: 3 gm, Carbohydrate: 19 gm, Dietary Fiber: 2 gm, Sodium: 160 mg

WHOLE WHEAT PIE CRUST *page 274*

Makes 8 servings; Serving size: 1 slice

Calories: 130, Total Fat: 6 gm, Saturated Fat: 0.5 gm, Monounsaturated Fat: 3.5 gm, Polyunsaturated Fat: 2 gm, Cholesterol: 0 mg, Protein: 3 gm, Carbohydrate: 17 gm, Dietary Fiber: 2 gm, Sodium: 150 mg

STRAWBERRY BANANA OAT BARS *page 275*

Makes 12 servings; Serving size: 1 bar

Calories: 100, Total Fat: 2.5 gm, Saturated Fat: 1 gm, Monounsaturated Fat: 1 gm, Polyunsaturated Fat: 0 gm, Cholesterol: 15 mg, Protein: 3 gm, Carbohydrate: 19 gm, Dietary Fiber: 3 gm, Sodium: 220 mg

DOUBLE CHOCOLATE CHEWS *page 276*

Makes 20 servings; Serving size: 1 cookie

Calories: 60, Total Fat: 2 gm, Saturated Fat: 1 gm, Monounsaturated Fat: 1 gm, Polyunsaturated Fat: 0 gm, Cholesterol: 0 mg, Protein: 2 gm, Carbohydrate: 13 gm, Dietary Fiber: 2 gm, Sodium: 70 mg

REFRESHING MIXED FRUIT KEBABS *page 278*

Makes 4 servings; Serving size: 1 kebab

Calories: 130, Total Fat: 0.5 gm, Saturated Fat: 0 gm, Monounsaturated Fat: 0 gm, Polyunsaturated Fat: 0 gm, Cholesterol: 0 mg, Protein: 2 gm, Carbohydrate: 34 gm, Dietary Fiber: 3 gm, Sodium: 5 mg

SWEET MANGO CRUMBLE *page 279*

Makes 18 servings; Serving size: 1 cup

Calories: 120, Total Fat: 2.5 gm, Saturated Fat: 0 gm, Monounsaturated Fat: 0.5 gm, Polyunsaturated Fat: 1.5 gm, Cholesterol: 0 mg, Protein: 3 gm, Carbohydrate: 22 gm, Dietary Fiber: 3 gm, Sodium: 10 mg

CINNAMON COFFEE CAKE *page 280*

Makes 12 servings; Serving size: 1 slice

Calories: 170, Total Fat: 7 gm, Saturated Fat: 1 gm, Monounsaturated Fat: 3 gm, Polyunsaturated Fat: 2 gm, Cholesterol: 15 mg, Protein: 3 gm, Carbohydrate: 24 gm, Dietary Fiber: <1 gm, Sodium: 240 mg

ALMOND COOKIE *page 282*

Makes 26 servings; Serving size: 1 cookie

Calories: 130, Total Fat: 5 gm, Saturated Fat: 0 gm, Monounsaturated Fat: 3 gm, Polyunsaturated Fat: 1.5 gm, Cholesterol: 5 mg, Protein: 2 gm, Carbohydrate: 19 gm, Dietary Fiber: <1 gm, Sodium: 70 mg

RICH FUDGE BROWNIES *page 283*

Makes 18 servings; Serving size: 1 brownie

Calories: 110, Total Fat: 4 gm, Saturated Fat: 0.5 gm, Monounsaturated Fat: 2 gm, Polyunsaturated Fat: 1 gm, Cholesterol: 10 mg, Protein: 2 gm, Carbohydrate: 17 gm, Dietary Fiber: <1 gm, Sodium: 10 mg

TASTY CHEESECAKE *page 284*

Makes 8 servings; Serving size: 1 slice

Calories: 300, Total Fat: 18 gm, Saturated Fat: 10 gm, Monounsaturated Fat: 0 gm, Polyunsaturated Fat: 0 gm, Cholesterol: 78 mg, Protein: 9 gm, Carbohydrate: 26 gm, Dietary Fiber: 1 gm, Sodium: 470 mg

LIGHT LEMON CAKE *page 286*

Makes 16 servings; Serving size: 1 piece

Calories: 100, Total Fat: 2 gm, Saturated Fat: 0 gm, Monounsaturated Fat: 1 gm, Polyunsaturated Fat: 0.5 gm, Cholesterol: 0 mg, Protein: 3 gm, Carbohydrate: 19 gm, Dietary Fiber: <1 gm, Sodium: 190 mg

BANANA CAKE *page 287*

Makes 16 servings; Serving size: 1 slice

Calories: 110, Total Fat: 0.5 gm, Saturated Fat: 0 gm, Monounsaturated Fat: 0 gm, Polyunsaturated Fat: 0 gm, Cholesterol: 0 mg, Protein: 3 gm, Carbohydrate: 25 gm, Dietary Fiber: 3 gm, Sodium: 220 mg

FRUIT COBBLER *page 288*

Makes 8 servings; Serving size: ½ cup

Calories: 170, Total Fat: 3 gm, Saturated Fat: 0.5 gm, Monounsaturated Fat: 1 gm, Polyunsaturated Fat: 1 gm, Cholesterol: 0 mg, Protein: 3 gm, Carbohydrate: 34 gm, Dietary Fiber: 3 gm, Sodium: 270 mg

CHERRY APPLE CRUMBLE *page 289*

Makes 10 servings; Serving size: ½ cup

Calories: 220, Total Fat: 7 gm, Saturated Fat: 0.5 gm, Monounsaturated Fat: 4 gm, Polyunsaturated Fat: 2 gm, Cholesterol: 0 mg, Protein: 4 gm, Carbohydrate: 38 gm, Dietary Fiber: 4 gm, Sodium: 55 mg

About the Author

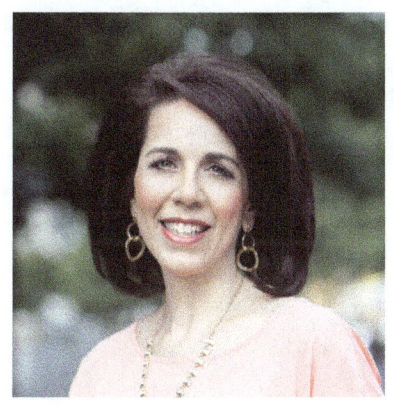

Bonnie R. Giller is a Registered and Certified Dietitian Nutritionist, Certified Diabetes Educator and Certified Intuitive Eating Counselor. She has her Master of Science degree in Clinical Nutrition and has worked in medical nutrition therapy and counseling for over 30 years.

Bonnie helps chronic dieters, emotional eaters, and people with medical conditions like diabetes, break free of the pain of dieting and get the healthy body and life they love. She does this by creating a tailored solution that combines three essential ingredients: a healthy mindset, caring support and nutrition education.

Using her signature Intuitive Eating Program, Bonnie helps her clients support and honor their mind and body. She works with adults, teens and youths, guiding them in changing their relationship with food and their body. The result is they make peace with food, enjoy guilt-free eating, and live a healthy life they love.

Bonnie is very passionate about helping her clients regain trust in themselves and their bodies so they can shift away from a diet mentality and learn to listen to their inner hunger and fullness signals. She is known for providing caring support and motivation as her clients reacquaint themselves with their inner wisdom.

Bonnie is the author of Passover the Healthy Way: Light, Tasty and Easy Recipes Your Whole Family Will Enjoy and My Supermarket Sidekick: Your Aisle-by-Aisle Shopping Guide.

Join the Free "Break the Spell of Diets in 3 Days" Online Experience at http://dietfreeradiantme.com/breakthespellexperience.

To learn more about intuitive eating, visit DietFreeRadiantMe.com.

For more information about nutrition therapy and lifestyle coaching, visit BRGHealth.com.

www.ingramcontent.com/pod-product-compliance
Lightning Source LLC
Chambersburg PA
CBHW081150290426
44108CB00018B/2494